For my husband Cian and our children
Sacha and Kim, with all my love

Emma Hannigan

All to Live For

Fighting Cancer. Finding Hope.

HACHETTE
BOOKS
IRELAND

First published in Ireland in 2017
by Hachette Books Ireland

1

The author and publishers take no responsibility for any of the tips contained in this book. Readers
should seek the advice of a professional in relation to any medical condition.

Cataloguing in Publication Data is available from the British Library

ISBN 978 1 4736 6170 7

Typeset in Bembo by Palimpsest Book Production Ltd, Falkirk, Stirlingshire

Printed and bound in Great Britain by
Clays Ltd, St Ives plc

Hachette Books Ireland's policy is to use papers that are natural, renewable and recyclable products
and made from wood grown in sustainable forests. The logging and manufacturing processes are
expected to conform to the environmental regulations of the country of origin.

Hachette Books Ireland
8 Castlecourt Centre
Castleknock
Dublin 15

An Hachette UK Company
Carmelite House
50 Victoria Embankment
London
EC4Y 0DZ

www.hachettebooksireland.ie

Contents

Prologue

My name is Emma Hannigan and I'm a shopaholic. I'm also a mother, wife, daughter, sister and friend. I regularly try on my own clothes and wonder how the hell I could ever have conceived of going out in public in a particular outfit.

Every day I intend drinking a minimum of eight glasses of water and eating at least the recommended five-a-day portions of fruit and vegetables. In reality, most days I drink too much coffee, not enough water and eat gout-encouraging amounts of chocolate. More and more, I catch glimpses of my own reflection and poke at my eyes, wondering where that new line sprang from. I'd love to have longer lashes, I hate my thighs and I always feel I could do with losing half a stone. Every week I vow I'll go to bed before nine o'clock at least once and have a wonderfully uninterrupted twelve-hour stretch of sleep. It never happens.

I'm always behind with the ironing, and the dirty clothes in my house seem to procreate in the wash-basket. For as long as I can remember, I've promised myself I'll get up that half-hour earlier so I don't have to rush out the door in the morning. Yet every day, I hit the snooze button and drift in and out of guilty yet delicious stolen moments of extra slumber. Inevitably someone eats breakfast in the car and the cat gets locked in the upstairs hallway and sets the house alarm off – again.

I thought I had my life fairly sorted. I thought I knew vaguely which direction I was heading in, give or take the odd unavoidable twist or turn. Towards the end of the summer of 2005, the rug was well and truly pulled from under me. Nothing could have prepared me for the road I was about to travel. In hindsight, I'm glad I didn't know what was ahead. In fact, I'd go so far as to say that, had I known what was coming, I wouldn't have thought I could cope. I wouldn't have credited myself with the strength to survive. As Garth

1

Brooks crooned in his song 'The Dance', I agree that our lives are indeed better left to chance. I think it's a good thing that we can't toddle down to the local shopping centre and buy a crystal ball.

Ten years ago, I can't say I would have been thrilled to have been given a detailed printout of my approaching ten-year plan. I think my immediate reaction would have involved phrases like 'Sod that' or 'You must be bloody joking – no thanks'. But, devoid of that crystal ball, I had to take events as they happened and, amazingly enough, I managed to deal with them.

In August 2005 I discovered I had a cancer-carrying gene called BRCA1. Between 2007 and 2015 I was diagnosed with and beat cancer eight times. I am currently battling for the tenth time. During the course of this book, I will try to take you on the journey that became my life at that tumultuous time.

A sense of humour was and still is one of the most important things in my life. That's what I would like to capture in the course of this tale – also, that there can be a sense of kinship and knowing you're not alone, even when you're faced with damn scary circumstances. That you can laugh even if you have cancer. That you don't have to feel isolated.

Cancer doesn't have to be a death sentence. I have been there and worn the T-shirt. Today, as I type these words to you, dear reader, I am undergoing treatment for the tenth time. Please don't throw the book away in fear! I'm only telling you it's been ten times because I need you to know that in spite of it hitting me so many times, I'm still here.

We all hear the bad stuff about cancer. We all know people die from this dreadful disease. All that I knew before I was diagnosed was negativity and finality where cancer was concerned.

I had no idea how many people survive. I had no concept of just how far medicine has progressed. I didn't realise that cancer isn't always a death sentence. Just because you're ill today, it doesn't mean you won't be fine again soon. The body is a complex and incredible machine, and it can bounce back from all sorts of traumas.

All I needed when I first started the cancer trail was someone to tell me I was going to be OK. That I could possibly survive. It was almost like I was emotionally thrust back to my schooldays, in the playground with a grazed knee. I needed a grown-up, or someone in the know, to hug me, then look me in the eye and say, 'It's going to be all right.'

My doctors were very positive, and for that I will be eternally grateful, but I guess I was looking for a non-medical person to tell me in plain English that it would all work out in the end. I wanted someone ordinary like me to tell me that I would survive. Obviously I'm not an oncologist. Nor am I able to jump off the pages of this book and analyse anybody's particular medical history. I can't offer a magic potion that will make cancer go away. I wish I could. But what I can tell you is that I'm still here in spite of ten diagnoses.

Against the odds, in spite of being very sick at one stage, I am alive to tell my tale. I had never been ill in my life before cancer crashed into my world. The only time I'd ever been in a hospital was to give birth to my two children. I didn't have any scars on my body, bar the small one on my knee from when, aged seventeen, I drove my moped into a wall at four in the morning.

I don't smoke, I'm not a heavy drinker, apart from the odd wedding, birthday party, New Year's Eve and on holidays – but that doesn't count, does it?

I eat a normal, healthy, balanced diet. I exercise a little, but only so I can eat more chocolate and still fit into my jeans.

I am a regular person. I am just like you.

I don't have special powers, have never seen a ghost. I'll hold my hands up and admit that I have serious trouble controlling my constant desire to go shopping. I don't believe in waiting for a rainy day – not that I'd wait long, living in Ireland! I think we should all live for the moment. I think we all have a right to happiness.

Cancer is not my favourite thing. I wouldn't recommend it to a friend. I believe there are other, pleasanter ways to build character. But, much as we all fear it, cancer and other horrible diseases are peppered through many of our lives. We can't stop most of them hitting us, but I am living proof that we can deal with them if they do. More than that, each and every one of us has the power still to be ourselves. Cancer doesn't have to take away the essence of who you are. It can shock the living daylights out of us. It can mean surgery and gruelling treatment. But for a rapidly growing number of patients, cancer can still be surmountable.

I might have had times when I was sick as a dog, weak as a kitten and looking like a gerbil (you'll understand later), but I have come out the other side. I am alive and on the road to recovery once more. I am confident that soon I will be able to fully enjoy my life again. I'm excited about having more energy and I know that will come in the not too distant future. My shopping habit is a lot worse, sadly. The guilt-factor area in my brain, which used to trigger easily after I'd been spending, has taken a huge hit. I now have an excuse to justify buying another pair of shoes.

I was really, really sick. I'm still a little bit sick, so I deserve a little treat.

Take it from me, I don't need any encouragement when it comes to shopping. Advertising works on me. I believe I'm worth it when celebrities tell me so. I get with the fever and I buy stuff. Whenever I can. Once the mortgage, bills and school fees are paid, I'm unstoppable.

There may never be a cure for my acute shopping addiction, but I hold out plenty of hope that the cure for cancer is within our grasp. In the last ten years alone, so many new forms of medication have been successfully adopted. I am only one person, a minuscule dot, in the sea of all this change, and I can see it.

I am currently on my third consecutive form of chemotherapy. The latest bout of cancer is being very rude and stubborn. But don't worry, this latest chemotherapy is working already so I have hope in my heart that I'll be better very soon.

There are positive advances all the time. So, if you're new to the cancer club, don't despair. I know it's not a popular club to be part of. Let's face it, given the choice, none of us would volunteer to join. But awful as it is, you still have a lot of choices. You can still control how you deal with your fight.

I knew the day I was diagnosed for the first time that I could either lie there and take it or shake myself up and fight it. I chose the latter. I vowed I would muster every shred of energy I could find to meet my challenge head-on.

I had my moments of fear and sadness. Of course I did. I'm not a robot. But most of the time I managed to keep my spirits high. I looked to my family and friends and drew all the positivity and joy I could from each of them. The cancer may have formed in my body, but I never allowed it to form in my mind.

I realised from day one that my spirit and wit couldn't be touched by sickness, unless I allowed it. There was never a hope in hell that I would let my physical sickness ruin my entire life. What's the point in being here on this earth if it's not going to be fun? I know every day can't be a party. I'm not a tree-hugging stick-waver who believes we should all stand and appreciate the shapes of the clouds and the colours of the rainbow. But I do like the idea that fairies might live in my garden. I know that laughter is the best medicine. I try to live for the moment and I never look back in anger. There's no point. I am living proof that there is life after cancer. Even if it keeps coming back, I'll just keep on crusading.

So, no more whispering. Laugh in the face of sickness, because there are no rules that state you have to lose the battle. Guess what? You might just win. I should know: so far I'm doing just that. If you have been diagnosed with cancer, or know someone who has, I have no doubt you're scared. I was too when I was diagnosed. But take my hand and, I promise you, it's possible to get through it. So put that shovel away. Stop lying on the patio to see if your body would fit underneath it. Don't dig that hole in your back garden just yet. Chin up, wig on – and don't forget your skin can absorb an astonishing amount of make-up.

Chapter 1

BRCA1

I never thought four little letters and one number could have such a sweeping effect. I am a positive person by nature, but for once I'm longing to be negative ...

Denise, my mum, comes from a family of nine children, eight of whom were girls. Amazingly, all of them live within a ten-kilometre radius of each other. So, as you can imagine, there has always been a strong female influence in my life.

My maternal grandmother was Austrian, so we called her 'Oma', the German for 'Granny'. My maternal grandfather was Scottish, so the family had a wonderful mix of dark-skinned, brunette, curly-haired divas and pale-skinned blondies. I am the Irish version of the latter. While my mum has green eyes, blond hair and skin that turns a deep golden colour in the sun, I am blond with skin like tracing paper that burns even in the shade. But I'm deft with a can of fake tan and know I can't leave the house without make-up or people will think I'm gravely ill. My natural skin tone is less pale and inter-esting, more akin to that of a corpse.

There has always been a history of cancer in my family. Oma's only sister, Anneliese, died on 6 October 1985 of ovarian cancer. In the years that followed, two of my aunts, Cathy and Ruth, were diagnosed with breast cancer. Following surgery, chemotherapy and radiation, both thankfully came through that. Alas several years later Ruth had a reocurrance, but yet again, she kicked cancer to touch. We've lost my only maternal uncle and two of my aunts to cancer.

I was only twelve when my aunts were having treatment, and I don't remember much about it. Nor was it widely discussed.

When Helen, another aunt, developed breast cancer, I was seventeen and instantly aware of it. She was a divorcée with three young children, Steffy, Robyn and Caleb. We were relatively close in age, so we'd always spent a lot of time together growing up. Helen was olive-complexioned, with tumbling chestnut curls and dancing eyes, and was knock-'em-dead stunning. She worked as an art teacher in a large girls' school and had an eye for style and a wicked sense of humour. In my mind's eye, I always see her as glamorous and dressed with flair, usually wearing deep red lipstick. I can still hear her infectious laugh.

Naturally we were all worried when Helen was diagnosed with breast cancer, but we hoped she would beat it. After all, both of my other aunts had. Sadly the cancer spread to her lungs. I vividly remember her and Mum talking in hushed tones in her house. Over the next couple of years Helen's health deteriorated. Her prognosis became bleak. She was taken to hospital and things went from bad to worse. We all knew she had a bad cough, but I don't remember the diagnosis ever being explained. All of us knew she was ill, but it became an unmentionable yet obvious fact that she was never coming out of hospital. I know it was a different time and the doctors even behaved differently from the way they do now – there were no open conversations about what was going on. So, much of Helen's illness was swept under the carpet.

Steffy, Robyn and I have discussed this at length. We know that all our family acted as they saw fit at the time, but none of us was taken aside and talked to. Nobody mentioned the big elephant in the room. Steffy was training to be a nurse at the time, so she knew better than any of us which way things were heading. I still recall Helen's illness being referred to as 'the big C'.

The disease had gone too far for the doctors to control it. Despite the best will in the world, on 15 May 1994, my beloved aunt Helen lost her fight with cancer. In the early hours of the morning, my father brought myself, Steffy and Robyn to see her for the last time. The image of her closed eyes and her face in eternal sleep is still vivid. Her hands were clasped across her chest, and she held a sprig of tiny white lilies-of-the-valley.

She looked relaxed, no longer in pain from the battle she had fought for so long. Her beautiful curls were long gone, ravaged by the endless chemotherapy. Her deep sallow glow had been replaced by a deathly pallor that all the medication had induced. But she looked at peace.

The only experience I'd had of death before this was when my best friend Anne-Marie had died in a car crash five years previously. Nicknamed Mim, she had been my closest friend since the age of three. We went to school together, played together at weekends and travelled together to Irish college the first time we went away from home. Her death in 1989 rocked me to the core. I was sixteen and thought we were immortal. Death had never entered the equation for either of us. I knew old people died, and although that was terribly sad, it seemed more acceptable.

When Anne-Marie and James, another classmate who was in the car, died, I thought I would never get over it. Cocooned by the loving and happy environment my parents had created for me, I found it almost impossible to fathom the pain of losing her. It was probably the harshest lesson and most difficult time of my life to date. We had done everything together. We chatted on the phone every night, planned everything around each other. Then she was gone. Quite simply, I needed to learn to live without her. At such a tender and tumultuous age, I had to deal with, attempt to understand and accept the notion of untimely death. Now, almost thirty years later, I still find the memory of that time gut-wrenching. I still miss Mim. I still talk to her a lot. I know she is with me and I draw comfort and solace from her spirit.

With Aunt Helen gone, Robyn came to live with us and joined our family as my sister. Steffy was still training to be a nurse, so she never actually lived with us, but I have always been close to her and consider her part of my immediate family. Caleb moved in with another aunt nearby. The only positive part of losing Helen was that I gained two sisters I adore in Steffy and Robyn, and I feel blessed to have them as a significant part of my life, as does my older brother Timmy – my bestest or worstest person in the world, depending on the mood of the moment.

Timmy was three and a half when I came to disrupt his world.

9

As my only sibling, he repeatedly reminded me that, in his humble opinion, 'Everything was fine until you came along.' In fairness to him, he did make several unsuccessful attempts to get rid of me before my first birthday. His first foiled endeavour involved pushing me down the very large steep hill near our house when I was less than a month old. My robust Silver Cross pram cushioned me until I landed unscathed in a pile of brambles. Like a cat, I seemed to have nine lives, even at that stage. Suffice to say, we were like all normal siblings, mostly in hate with one another, only forming allegiances when other children threatened to biff us. It was OK for us to kill each other, but the privilege didn't extend to others. That sense of fun – and the knowledge that there is always a reason to smile – has carried me through even the roughest times.

Ten years after Helen's death, in March 2005, our family was approached by the National Centre for Medical Genetics at the Children's Hospital in Crumlin, Dublin. Due to the significant incidence of cancer in the family, they asked if any of Mum's generation would be willing to put themselves forward for testing. A cancer-carrying gene called BRCA1 had been discovered. This stands for 'breast cancer one'. If we were to discover we carried the gene, the testing centre would provide us with the information we needed to be able to handle it.

This was well before Angelina Jolie discovered she carries the gene. So there was no media coverage or hype, and we knew nothing about it and had to learn, fast.

So, what would a gene-positive result signify? Basically, it would mean we were at an increased risk of developing breast cancer and/ or ovarian cancer. The odds were high too. It would mean an 85 per cent chance that breast cancer would develop, and a 50 per cent chance of ovarian cancer.

This information met a mixed reaction among my family members. Some of us wanted to be tested and needed to know either way. Others wanted nothing to do with the whole thing, feeling they would rather continue with their lives just as they had before – going for the 'ignorance-is-bliss' option. Although the latter wasn't for me, I could appreciate why some felt they didn't want to be privy to that kind of knowledge.

For me, the decision was a no-brainer. I was the mother of two small children, and there was also my husband, Cian. I met Cian on 22 February 1997 when I was twenty-three, working in Hard Metal and studying at night to be a beautician. Before you think I'd lost all sense of reality, Hard Metal was my parents' engineering company, rather than a blacked-out bus with Ozzy Osbourne lookalikes strumming electric guitars and head-banging while making menacing noises. I was at POD nightclub, in Dublin city centre, with a couple of friends, clearing my head with gin and shots of tequila, the night Cian and I met.

Even though I was only twenty-three, I'd had a run of bad luck on the boyfriend front and had come to the conclusion that I would be better off as a nun, a lesbian or a hermit – but Cian and I gravitated towards one another. We recognised each other from school, through a fog of dry ice, amid flashing lights and many gallons of alcohol on the dance floor. We clicked immediately. There were no agendas, no mind games. Within two months of meeting, we moved in together. Just over a year later, we were married. Our wedding was, as the cliché goes, one of the best days of my life. I loved the build-up, and although I waited for the meltdown and stress that others had warned me about, they didn't happen. On our first wedding anniversary, I was already three months pregnant with our son, Sacha. Eighteen months later our daughter Kim graced us with her presence, to complete our family.

I loved them so much that I would go anywhere and do anything to entertain them and keep them busy and happy. If this monster was lurking in my genes, I needed to know. If not for me, for Sacha, Kim and Cian. I owed it to them to do everything in my power to fight to stay alive.

Step one didn't involve me directly. The rules with the test were this: for me to be tested, my mother had to be gene-positive. Mum is one of the most chilled-out people I know. She is serene without being submissive and has effortless style and elegance. She balances her time brilliantly between office work, gardening, swimming, horse riding, walking dogs, cooking, shopping, being a wife for more than forty years, mother and Oma – among other things, of course. I was lucky enough to have ten cousins when I was younger, who would roll up and play on a regular basis: our house was always heaving with friends and everyone was welcome. Mum liked to cook and bake, and I can't remember a time when I didn't know how to make a pot of meatballs or an apple crumble. We always found something to laugh about. When I picture my mum in my mind's eye, she is always smiling.

If Mum was clear of the BRCA1 gene, that was it – the buck would stop there. But she had a 50 per cent chance of having it. Without being too scientific and running the risk of boring you to tears, this is how it works.

We all have a pair of genes, apart from the denim kind. To help you with the imagery, picture a pair of trousers. In order to make up the full pair, one leg comes from our mother, and the other comes from our father. Hey presto! A pair of trousers or, more specifically, genes.

In my case, my maternal grandmother had one normal leg of genes and one defective leg. If she had passed on the defective leg to my mum, she, too, would be 'gene positive'.

The physical ritual for testing is simple. It involves a routine blood sample being sent to a genetic testing laboratory in England. The scientists break down the blood and search certain points of the genetic chain for defects. The entire process, from having the blood sample taken to finding out the result, is estimated at six weeks.

'What do you think?' Mum asked me.

'I don't want to push you into doing anything you're not comfortable with, but I really want to know. Forewarned is forearmed, is it not?' I reasoned.

Having mulled it over for a few days, Mum decided she would put herself forward for testing. 'I have a 50 per cent chance of being fine, so it's better to just go for it and find out, isn't it?' she said. 'If I don't have the gene, I could put myself through years of needless worry.'

'Absolutely. And if you don't have it, neither do I, so that'll be the end of the line as far as we're concerned,' I encouraged her.

Once we had made the decision to go ahead, it all moved swiftly. As our family had been approached, we had a green light and a direct route to the entire process. We got an appointment within days and I accompanied my mum to the children's hospital. As we walked along the clammy corridors, we averted our eyes and hearts from the pain and suffering we witnessed at every turn. In my mind, there is nothing more heartbreaking than an ill child.

We met Nuala Cody, a gentle and gorgeous genetics expert. She explained that the gene was rare but it held potentially scary consequences. We were nervous and, of course, hoping Mum would get a negative result, but determined to know the truth.

'If you want to wait a while and think about taking the test, there's no hurry,' Nuala explained.

But Mum had made up her mind. She knew I was desperate to find out if I carried the gene. She was my stepping-stone and she was doing it partly for me. I am thankful to this day that she took that decision.

Nuala directed us to the phlebotomy, or blood-testing, department, where a small glass tube of Mum's blood was sealed and sent on its merry way. Our family's journey with BRCA1 had begun.

Chapter 2

Mamma Mia!

As a mother, I would always wish to take my children's pain if I could. Being a daughter is no different. I want to take my mother's pain now too. If I buy enough steroids on eBay, how long would it take me to resemble Hercules?

Other than when I was pregnant, I don't remember a six-week period taking so long. We hadn't discussed the process outside the immediate family. I'm the worst person at keeping big things to myself. When we were younger, we were always encouraged to speak our minds and never forced to do anything we didn't like. I don't remember being made to feel like my opinion didn't count.

The older I get, the more I realise just how lucky we were during those childhood and teenage years. That's not to say I don't stay quiet if a friend tells me a secret – that's a different kettle of fish. I would always keep someone else's secrets, but my own are another matter entirely. This was a potentially huge thing, yet there was no point in telling everyone, should it not become relevant to us.

As a result, I was flying around, trying to keep my mind active and not think about the test result. Easier said than done. At this stage Sacha and Kim were five and four years old respectively. Sacha had started big school and Kim was in her second year at Montessori – I had got myself through the full-time baby-minding stage and was ready to become an upwardly mobile yummy mummy. I had been working at Hard Metal since before Sacha was born and was at the point in my life where I could finally look at devoting more time to my career.

After I'd finished school, I had done Darina Allen's cookery course in Cork, before spending two years cooking in the main kitchen of Ballymaloe House, so, as my office work was only part-time, I took on a few small catering jobs, private dinner parties and freezer cooking, that sort of thing. I had joined a health club and tried to convince myself I could get to like exercise. I'd bought a trendy, stretchy Barbie-goes-to-the-gym outfit with matching trainers and little socks with sparkly pom-poms at the heel. I even managed to attend the gym and do my recommended and customised workout, ooh, probably six times before I admitted to myself that the gym and I were never going to feel the love for one another. I did use the pool regularly and resigned myself to the fact that swimming (slowly and without a huge amount of finesse) was the only form of physical exercise I could force myself to pursue. I discovered that the toned, tanned, hair-swishing yummy-mummy look was bloody difficult to achieve, never mind keep up, but over those weeks I did anything to try to keep myself calm.

I was so edgy, I felt I was in danger of blurting things to random strangers.

'Good morning, nice day,' said the postman.

I'd have to force myself not to shout, 'We might have a deadly cancer gene, but apart from that, it's business as usual around here.'

Friends asking a run-of-the-mill question like 'Any news?' or even 'How's tricks?' caused me untold inner turmoil.

'Nothing springs to mind,' I'd lie.

Inside I'd be screaming: 'Yes, I have news. Mum and I might be walking time bombs, ready to explode into a massive cancer tumour with eyes.'

Or even, 'Tricks are damned sticky, to be frank. I could be in an 85-per-cent danger bracket – doesn't get much bloody dicier than that, does it?'

Instead I thanked God for the invention of the telephone and the fact that no one could see my face as I sidestepped the truth and pretended things were hunky dory.

It became more and more difficult to talk about teething problems and nappy rash. When one distressed pal, then the mother of a two-and-a-half-year-old, rang to ask my advice on her little boy who had overheard a man shouting 'Piss off' at a dog, and was now repeating the phrase to everyone from her mother-in-law to the lady at crèche, I couldn't sympathise.

'I don't blame him shouting "Piss off ". He's probably so thrilled to have words to verbalise how he feels that he wants to say it to everyone who annoys him.' I wished I could shout 'Piss off' to everyone I met.

During that six-week stint, sometimes I would convince myself that Mum didn't have the gene. That we would walk away from the whole notion, exhaling and thanking our lucky stars that we were free of the potential risk. More often, I heard a niggling voice whispering in my head, 'Mum will be gene-positive, and so will I.'

Eventually a phone call came. Nuala wanted to see Mum. She had the result. We arranged to attend the hospital the following day. Dad offered to come, but Mum and I felt we wanted to do it together.

'Denise, I have your result here. I am sorry to say you have indeed tested positive for the BRCA1 gene.' Nuala was gentle and sympathetic. The silence in the room was deafening.

'I didn't think it was going to be positive,' Mum whispered in utter disbelief.

'I did.' I'd said it before I could think. 'Sorry, Mum. I didn't mean to sound callous or cold, but I think I knew.'

'The particular mutation that your family carries is called the Ashkenazi Jewish mutation.'

'My mother was of Jewish decent,' Mum explained to Nuala. 'Her parents fled Austria towards the end of the Second World War. Her mother was Jewish, so that would explain the connection.'

'Are you OK?' Nuala leaned forward and waited for Mum to gather herself.

'I'm actually stunned, to be honest.' Mum was choked. We hugged silently and let the news sink in.

I might not have been speaking, but my head was working overtime. I was trying to run through all the things I'd read on the Internet.

Nuala chatted to us and explained the options available to Mum.

First, she could be monitored. This meant yearly mammograms, six-monthly breast examinations with a specialist breast surgeon, transvaginal scanning of the ovaries and regular self-checking. The second option was surgery: a double mastectomy, to remove all breast tissue, and an oophorectomy, or removal of both ovaries and the Fallopian tubes. Mum had had a full hysterectomy several years previously, so she was one down on the operating stakes.

Nuala gave us printouts of all the information we'd discussed, with a list of surgeons who might be able to help us further. Wasting no time, we contacted one immediately. Within weeks, Mum had an appointment with a specialist who knew about BRCA1.

'The fact that you have no ovaries reduces your risk, Denise. This means the ovarian cancer risk is down from 50 per cent to less than 5 per cent,' the surgeon explained. 'Also, the removal of the hormones reduces the risk of breast cancer. So you are no longer at 85 per cent risk either. The good news is your age. The fact that you are heading for sixty means mammograms are a good and viable option for you.'

I was terrified for her. In fact, if it had been possible to remove the defective gene from my mum and pass it on to me, I would gladly have had it. I hated the thought of her getting ill. I had to block the memory of Helen when she was dying, and not allow myself to place my own mother in that hypothetical situation.

I had to get a grip on my emotions. I had to remain calm and stop my mind wandering off on tangents where I conjured up all the worst-case scenarios known to woman.

We left the hospital that day with information overload. Mum went home to break the news to my father, and I went home to tell Cian.

Before walking into the house I sat in the car and, for some bizarre reason, memories of our wedding day flooded my mind. We'd had a string quartet in the gardens of the hotel, with blazing sunshine – one of my angels up above must have kindly organised that. I have a penchant for angels. I like to think that we all have at least one watching over us at all times. I'm not obsessed with this notion, it's more like a warm, fuzzy thought that washes over me from time to time. A bagpiper played Cian and me into the function room for dinner, where two hundred and fifty inebriated and rather rowdy guests clapped and whooped. Then one of our oldest family friends, John Terry, a.k.a. Hurricane Johnny and the Jets, belted out a couple of hours of kick-ass rock-'n'-roll numbers. The final nail in the coffin, which was supposed to rid the room of anyone over the age of twenty-five, was Mr Spring, a.k.a. Timmy, my DJ brother, on the decks. But seeing as it was our parents and their equally insane friends, they decided not only to stay until five in the morning, but to dance on the tables for good measure.

I did get a raised eyebrow at the dry-cleaner's the day I brought in my wedding dress. 'There are actual footprints on this. Were you wearing it or using it as a floor covering?'

Cian and I went to St Lucia for our honeymoon. The all-inclusive resort offered all-day cocktails, complimentary massages, facials, salt rubs, full body wraps and an extensive range of water sports. Our marriage survived the honeymoon. We learned a lot about each other. Cian knew for certain that I was never going to share his love of all things sporty. More than that, I had managed to demonstrate in no uncertain terms that I had the sporting aptitude and ability of a brick. After a painful two-hour excursion to a local Caribbean market, where Cian looked like he was being physically and mentally tortured, I knew he was allergic to shopping.

Since our honeymoon, we have successfully managed to pursue and enjoy our diverse activities while maintaining communication. We have matured and changed together, never losing sight of who we are as individuals.

I knew our relationship was steadfast and strong. We'd come through the first few years of Sacha and Kim's lives. I was in the very fortunate position of being able to stay at home with our children while they were babies, but now they were in school, it was supposed to be the start of a new chapter for us. We had plans for our little family. As they grew older we would take them on long-haul flights across the world, and Cian was looking forward to encouraging them to do sport with him – God bless him. We were on the cusp of moving on to the next exciting phase of our lives.

As I climbed out of the car and walked in the front door of our house that day in 2005, I knew I was presenting Cian with a totally different pitch. The defective gene, if I carried it, was going to change the course of our road. I knew I was asking him to come with me on a different route from the one we'd assumed we'd travel. A new sign was being erected for us.

I showed Cian the information the genetic-testing people had provided. Over a glass of wine and several hours of conversation, we tried to digest the implications that could be about to impact on us all. Cian was calm and supportive from the outset. He has always encouraged and listened to me on important issues. The rest of the time, he doesn't hear 90 per cent of what I say – especially if it involves a dinner he doesn't want to go to, gossip or girly stuff.

Just like any new situation, the beginning was the worst part. We had to work through that transition from blissful ignorance into a new zone of scary territory. We needed to process our facts and weigh up the options. Mum needed to figure out what she was comfortable with and what would afford her the best peace of mind in going forward.

We all needed to pull together as a family.

After many hours of discussion and tossing ideas back and forth, Mum and Dad decided the best option for her was regular screening. We needed to find the right professionals to mind Mum and provide her with the best chance of a positive outcome, whatever might arise. She was fortunate to find a wonderful consultant oncologist who added regular MRI scans of the breast to the monitoring plan. To this day, Mum is still being monitored and thankfully has not had cancer. This is a really important fact to note. My mother is gene-positive. Her mother before her was gene-positive. So far my mother is still cancer-free. My grandmother never developed cancer. She died of other causes in January 2009, but she never had cancer. So even if you or someone you know has been diagnosed as a carrier of the BRCA1 gene, it doesn't necessarily mean you will get cancer. I know the odds are high, but someone has to make up the 15 per cent of people who remain healthy!

Chapter 3

Blood, Sweat and Tears

I feel like it's my turn to walk the plank. Will Tinkerbell please swoop down and save me? I never harboured a desire to be a superhero. But, right now, I'm hankering after that cloak and the Wonder Woman hot pants – even though I utterly hate my thighs.

Once Mum was sorted and we knew the plan of action she was going to follow, the baton was passed to me. If my mother had the gene, I had a 50 per cent chance of having it also. I had a decision to make. Would I go for the test? It was all very fine and dandy to say I would when it wasn't my turn – we're all great at being brave and expressing opinions about other people's situations. When the limelight shone on me, there was nowhere to hide. This was it.

Prior to that time, I'd never thought of myself as a particularly brave person. I wasn't well-versed in the whole hospital scene, apart from for my pregnancies. Letting you in on a little secret, I wasn't very good at it. If there had been any possible way of getting someone else to do pregnancy and birth for me, I would've gone for it. The day I found out I was pregnant with our first child, I sat with shaking hands staring at the urine-soaked stick and promptly burst out crying. After that, I spent the entire nine months wide awake. Fear crept in and took over my brain. Sheer terror made me contemplate every possible defect the baby might be born with, ranging from two heads to missing limbs, depending on that day's level of neurosis. I bolstered my own insane inner thoughts with other people's by obsessively logging on to some helpful and plenty of dreadful websites.

Many women I encountered during those months of rapid physical expansion took on an odd sort of misty look and did that vice grip on my forearm as they told me how much they'd loved being pregnant. That they'd never felt healthier. That their hair had shone, their skin had glowed and they'd had the energy of ten triathletes.

I, on the other hand, gained five stone with our son Sacha and four and a half with our daughter Kim. I had raised blood pressure, swelling due to water retention and protein in my urine. I looked and felt like a raw, overstuffed white pudding with eyes. There were no shining locks or glowing skin for me. My hair fell out in clumps and I had to shuffle in for the delivery wearing my father's slippers. I was so fat I even went up a shoe size. A member of the looking-into-the-misty-middle-distance club? Not me. Sorry if I'm raining on the pregnancy parade, but I found it hideous. All that banging my bump off cupboards and getting stuck in soft chairs. (If you take no other pregnancy tips, remember this one: don't ever sit in a beanbag. You'll have to wait for someone to hire a cherry-picker to lift you out.)

Luckily I didn't die during the birth of either of my children. Yes, I was that neurotic. I had decided that, although for centuries other women had managed this allegedly natural act, I would be somehow exempt. Nor did I produce a multi-headed alien.

I did the natural childbirth thing by mistake. It was so damn quick, the trainee midwife had only managed to untangle the oxygen mask and hook it up to the can of loopy-juice before it was all over. I did protest and ask for the epidural anyway, but my gynaecologist wasn't having any of it: you could only have the drugs before you gave birth. There was no offer of a go on the laughing gas by way of compensation either.

I was proud beyond words that I had managed to conceive, grow and give birth to two healthy children. But I still didn't consider myself brave. At any given time, I would have traded all my favourite possessions to get out of childbirth, and I spent the entire duration of both pregnancies drenched in fear. So, when it came to dealing with a possible genetic defect, the thought of so much as a blood test didn't fill me with joy. But any hesitation I felt was wiped clean away with just a glimpse of my children. I hadn't expanded to the size of a hippo twice, and stayed awake for eighteen months filling my head with nightmare scenarios, to back out now. My two babies were my heart and soul personified and, come hell or high water, I was going to do my utmost to stay around to raise them.

I felt strongly that what I was being faced with was positive. How many people have the chance to find out if they're likely to get cancer? I was being offered the opportunity to gain that very important knowledge. Rather than the whole notion filling me with fear, I felt empowered. I was going to grasp that chance with both hands. I was also aware that when Kim is older, this issue will become relevant for her. Once she reaches the age of eighteen, she will be entitled to have genetic testing carried out, should she choose to do so. Like I had, she will have a 50 per cent chance of being a gene carrier.

I phoned the genetic testing centre and made my appointment. As I stood in the hall there, waiting to have my blood test done, waves of nerve-twanging trepidation crescendoed through me. I was nervous, of course I was, but I felt like I was taking control. For me that was the most important factor.

On that fateful day in the hospital, 5 July 2005, I think some of Helen's courage had somehow crept into me by osmosis. As I sat and had the small amount of blood extracted from my arm, I vowed that I would follow through the entire process with gusto. Mum had accompanied me. We have always been extremely close, but that time in our lives without doubt bonded us more tightly than I'd ever thought possible. She knew exactly how I was feeling because she'd been in my shoes only weeks previously.

Before I could go wholeheartedly into the Braveheart thing, I had to feel a bit sorry for myself. The blood test left me with a dead arm, and mentally I felt like I'd donated enough blood to supply the entire blood bank of *M.A.S.H.*, should they ever decide to do a new series.

Once I'd had a can of Diet Coke and consumed my own body-weight in chocolate, I was ready to stand up and fight, should my blood test yield a positive result. I braced myself and began to put on my armour inside my head.

As I sit typing today and think back to how I felt at that time, I realise that I had already made my peace with the situation. Deep down, I had already accepted that I had the defective gene. Perhaps that was a protection mechanism, to help with the impact. But, like those months when I was pregnant, I did more lying awake for hours in the darkness of night. I pounded the prom at Bray seafront during the day and mulled it all over in my mind. I came to terms with a positive result before the people at the lab in England had even taken delivery of my blood.

Chapter 4

Waiting to Exhale

Whether it's positive or negative, I need the guessing to stop. Have you ever realised you've been mentally holding your breath for a long time?

Patience is not a virtue I possess. I've never been good as a sitting duck. From the time I did my final state exams in school, I've always been on the lookout for something new and exciting to fill my time. As I mentioned before, I started my working life as a chef under the capable guidance of Darina and Myrtle Allen at Ballymaloe House. It's a fantastic life skill to have. Everyone needs to eat, so the years I spent working in a commercial kitchen and running my own catering business will always stand to me. A neck injury from a car rear-ending me forced me to change career. I had very limited knowledge of computers, so I took myself off to do a general business course in Dublin city centre. To say that I was not naturally suited to sit for long periods being quiet is putting it mildly. To alleviate the boredom, I wisely used the time outside the course schedule to go out until the small hours dancing and being debauched.

The lack of sleep, abundance of alcohol and reluctance to learn about business started me on the road to drinking strong coffee. I had never tasted tea or coffee until then. To this day the smell of tea makes me gag. The college I was attending was a stone's throw from Bewley's coffee house, where they used to supply us with freshly brewed, tar-strength coffee. At first I used to make a face like a professional gurner as I drank shots of the black liquid. A determined personality, I weighed up the pros and cons. Either I got kicked out of business school for snoring in class or I got used to downing coffee and survived. (Going to bed at a reasonable hour or spending less time on the batter was obviously out of the question.) Thinking about it in a logical manner, I figured that if I could drink tequila without vomiting, I could also master coffee. I tried the milk and sugar accompaniment and found that horrific. Black and strong was the way to go. It gave me that hairs-on-your-chest sensation. It was so vile to my palate that I convinced myself it must be good for me. To my delight, it kept me awake and cut out the rude awakenings I kept suffering at the hands of my irate teacher.

'So sorry to wake you, Emma, but you're not supposed to sleep blatantly while the rest of us are attempting to learn.'

'Sorry, Miss, I'm awake now.'

I'd have to peel my face off the keyboard and hope to God I hadn't dribbled into the computer, lining myself up for electrocution and sudden death by my own saliva.

At the end of the three-month course, I knew how to type, answer phones, do basic computing and book-keeping, lay out business letters and lots of other very useful officey things. Most of all, I knew how to stay awake after two hours' sleep – a handy tool to have, no matter where life takes you.

I put my course to use and tried to do the nine-to-five thing at Hard Metal.

The lack of movement and buzz began to get to me. I decided to go to college at night and learn to be a beauty therapist. That unwittingly brought out the sadist in me. I had a preconceived idea that it would be about pampering and make-up, with a bit of nail painting thrown in. In reality it predominantly involved hair and blackhead removal. But that was fine by me. I loved the instant results of waxing and the immediate glow that clients emanated after a facial. All right, I'm lying. I enjoyed pouring molten wax on people and ripping it off. And the notion that I could get paid for inflicting such pain? Result.

I also recorded my first song, courtesy of that course. Well, there was no actual music involved – instead it featured me droning the names, origins and mechanics of all the muscles. I had to learn these, and as they all have convoluted Latin names, most of which sound like a very drunk person invented them, I couldn't get them into my head. I spoke them into a tape recorder and made myself listen to them on my car stereo as I sat in traffic.

You know the way people tell you that all education helps to shape you? That doing any course or form of study will always stand to you? Well, my diverse career paths all served a purpose while I waited for the results of my blood test. Just as I had while Mum's blood was on its little journey, I proceeded to go into personal overdrive. I invited friends over, waxed any fuzzy parts they offered and fed them home-baked goods with strong coffee. When I was on the brink of driving myself and all those around me insane, something clicked in my head.

For crying out loud, I'd lived through two pregnancies and eaten enough burgers to put Elvis to shame. Afterwards, I'd pounded the pavement and inflicted my swimming-togs-clad body on the local pool to beat that five stone off me. I wasn't going to waste all that pain by dying. If knowing about BRCA1 could forewarn me of possible danger ahead, I was going to strike out and take positive action.

Cian, like a lot of men, is of the opinion that one should deal only with facts. Hypothetical situations carry no whack with him. So, until I'd had the test, he didn't want to enter into discussion about it too much. Yes, he'd listened when I presented him with the information in the beginning. Yes, he'd phoned constantly the day I went for the blood test. Yes, he asked me plenty of times if I was coping. But, no, he didn't want to talk about it incessantly, from the moment I woke until the second I went to the Land of Nod each night.

'If and when we have to face this conundrum, I'll give it all my attention. Otherwise, let's not talk about it non-stop.'

If I'm making him sound unfeeling or callous, he most certainly isn't. Cian is one of those rare people who hates bitching or back-biting. If he has something to say, he'll say it to your face. You always know where you stand with him. He sees the best in people, and unless you do something to really piss him off, he'll like you. But he is a man. Fact. So he doesn't understand my need to shop – he cannot comprehend why anyone needs more than one pair of shoes. He will never get why I feel the need to talk for an hour on the phone to a friend I've just spent all morning with. But when, at long last, the call came from Nuala, Cian immediately volunteered to accompany me.

Just like before, an appointment was set up for the following morning. I was glad Cian was going to be there, so he could chat to Nuala if necessary. If the result was positive, I wanted him to be able to ask questions for himself. There's nothing like getting direct information from an expert.

Cian and I sat in the hospital corridor where I'd waited with Mum. We were there for about ten minutes. It felt like a week. The pale blue walls echoed the cold feelings that were lurching in the pit of my stomach.

As if in some subconscious reaction to the serious note of the day, I'd worn a pink glittery T-shirt, stark white jeans with crystals on the backside and bubblegum-coloured ballerina shoes. All I was missing was the Cosmopolitan cocktail and the flashing disco boppers.

'Do you think I might have gone a bit *Sex and the City* with the outfit?' I asked.

'When have you been any different?' Cian smiled.

'Emma, step this way.' Nuala appeared and gestured to us to follow her.

'OK?' Cian squeezed my hand as we both took a deep breath.

'Bring it on.' I nodded firmly as I followed Nuala.

'Come on in.' Nuala smiled warmly at us both.

I introduced Cian and we exchanged pleasantries, but not for long. I couldn't stand it any longer. 'I apologise if I sound curt, Nuala. Please put me out of my misery. I now know I'm the most impatient person on the planet.' I smiled to show I wasn't angry, just anxious.

'Emma, I'm sorry to say that you are gene-positive too.'

The geneticist was an exceptionally serene and gentle person. If she could have willed my genetic disposition to be different, she would have.

I swallowed. I closed my eyes for a second longer than necessary. This revelation meant I had an 85 per cent chance of developing breast cancer and a 50 per cent chance of developing ovarian cancer.

Unless I did something about it. I didn't need reminding that both types of cancer had already claimed Helen and Anneliese.

I don't remember there being a loud noise or any audible click, but the gears changed inside my head. My brain went from live-mode to survive-mode. From that moment on, I knew I was going to do everything in my power to stay alive.

In most situations life has thrown at me, I will find something to laugh about. I will pick on the most bizarre aspect and turn it into a joke. That day, I was fresh out of one-liners.

Cian asked a few questions and accepted the same information pack that Mum had been given a few months previously.

'Call me if I can be of any further assistance,' Nuala offered.

We emerged from the hospital into the August sunshine. I handed Cian the car-parking ticket and stood like I was made of plaster of Paris. He took the car key from my hand and I followed him to the car. We hugged, then wordlessly got in and drove home. I would love to say that we smiled at each other as poignant songs like 'I Will Survive' or 'Stayin' Alive' just happened to burst forth from the radio. But the reality was that we were both trying to digest the facts and come to terms with what should happen next.

Although many people have commented to me that they would have crumbled when told they were gene-positive, I felt an odd satisfaction. I had known I would carry the gene. I was glad that my strong hunch had been right. In a funny way, it gave me self-confidence about my own body. Not in a how-to-look-good-naked type of way, but in a more I-am-in-tune-with-my-own-workings sort of way.

How did I feel, knowing I had an inbuilt predisposition to get cancer?

In a word – terrified. The way I saw it, I had a choice of two roads to take.

The first involved wallowing and feeling sorry for myself. I could have gone on a personal rant about how unfair it was that our family had been cursed with this damned gene. Or I could do an ostrich and stick my head in the sand. But what was the point of that?

The second road involved embracing the positive elements of my life and going for it.

What's positive about being diagnosed with BRCA1, I hear you cry? Plenty. I had something vital: information. I'd had a warning. Put it this way, if your entire house must go on fire, wouldn't you be eternally grateful if you had even ten minutes' notice, so you could run around and free all your family? Imagine if you had twenty minutes' notice and could also rescue all your cherished photographs, plus your other most precious belongings. Imagine if you had an hour's notice. You'd do a lot, wouldn't you?

Well, to me, being told I was gene-positive gave me that crucial notice. It afforded me the time to take a deep breath and decide what to do, with calm clarity.

In September 2005, shortly after I had been diagnosed with the BRCA1 gene, I attended the children's hospital in Dublin once again to get information detailing my options.

I had Sacha and Kim with me, and as we waited in the corridor, with the murals on the walls and the animal-shaped bins, I scanned the chipped bookshelf containing curled-at-the-edges, battered books.

'Don't touch the books,' I whispered discreetly, not wanting to offend anyone.

'Why?' they chorused very loudly.

'Just in case they're carrying disease. They look old, and not everybody washes their hands, you know.'

Of course, that prompted giggles and the perfect opening for a gleeful conversation about 'wee' and 'poo'.

They moved on to the only other form of in-house entertainment, which was one of those blocks of wood with a maze of wiggly wires banged into it. The object of the game appeared to involve threading a few beads along the wiggles from one side to the other.

'What's this supposed to do?' Sacha was unimpressed.

'Just what you're doing – maybe you could time each other,' I suggested brightly. They had zero interest in that idea and instead started trying to vandalise the poor toy. In fairness to it, Bob the Builder, or whoever had constructed it, had done a fabulous job and they didn't succeed. Under normal circumstances I would've hissed at them that they were to stop immediately and come and sit down. I was very strict about manners and respecting other people's things. But that day I wouldn't have cared if they'd thrown the toy through the window. Discipline seemed unimportant, and besides there was nobody else in the corridor.

To prevent myself melting in the dense heat of the place, I removed as much clothing as was legally allowed and meandered towards a glass panel at the end of the corridor. It was being used to display artwork drawn by sick children, presumably during art therapy. Beneath it, the hospital had placed a collection bin, with a sign stating that any donation, large or small, would be gratefully received.

Most of the children had drawn around either their hand or foot, cut out the shape, coloured it brightly and glued it onto a piece of stiff card. Only one cut-out had writing underneath it. I had to stoop and squint to read it. The writing was faded, and although it was bockety and spidery, the words chilled me to the bone. It read: 'Help me to die, I am suffering. Katie, age 7.'

Needless to say, after emptying the contents of my handbag into the collection, I scuttled back down the corridor and pulled both my children into an embrace.

'Why are you looking sad, Mummy?' Sacha asked.

I struggled to speak. 'I just read a lovely message that a little girl who wasn't well wrote.'

'Is she better now?' Kim looked very worried. 'Where is she?' Breaking free from my arms, she ran towards the glass panel to see.

'She's not there, Kim. She's in a much nicer place than here,' I answered.

I have drawn from that defining moment so many times over the last few years. Remember the old-fashioned saying 'There's always someone worse off than yourself'? OK, I get that this is meant to strike a chord with us all. Now, maybe I'm a terrible person, because before I had that moment of clarity, that saying used to bring out a sort of inner violence in me. It made me think, 'Oh, just sod off.' I honestly thought it was the type of thing grumpy and bitter old people said, as they wagged a wizened finger at young kids, willing them to stop having fun. But that day, in that hospital, wham! I got it.

A new internal vigour engulfed me. It was like a driving force, pushing me forward and willing me on. I collected the list of surgeons and medical centres I could approach. I was determined to take control of my situation and to use the information I had been given in the most constructive way possible.

That defining moment, which hit me like a bolt out of the blue, has bolstered me many times over the last few years. The simple yet heartbreaking words of a small child suffering conjure up an image that I know I couldn't cope with. As long as my children are safe and healthy, I will always fight the good fight to stay with them. I would gladly accept any surgery, illness or pain in their place. That day at the children's hospital especially, I was glad it was me who was having to weigh up options and make decisions about my own body, not one of the children's. I cannot imagine how families cope with the loss of a child. It quite simply doesn't bear thinking about.

We drove home, and when Sacha asked if we could stop and buy chips, I said yes. It might annoy him hugely when he's older, but if he'd asked me to buy him the entire aisle of boys' things in the toy shop that day, I would have done it. Lucky for all concerned, the credit card stayed safely in my purse and I had two very excited, clapping children for the price of a bag of chips!

Chapter 5

Come on Down, the Price is Right

Today, Emma, you have won a choice of prizes beyond your wildest dreams. Take a look at your showcase. You could stand to win breast cancer – and that's not all, we could throw in a nice dose of ovarian cancer to accompany it. All you have to do is just sit and do nothing and all this could be yours …

Life still had to carry on, even though I was facing this enormous, life-altering time. I still had to go to my part-time job, be the housekeeper, pot-washer, cook, wife and mother. One part of me wanted to hide in the basement and use every moment of every day to gather information on BRCA1. Another part of me was truly grateful that I had a family to mind, a house to run and work to go to.

The children had no idea of what was going on, and as far as they were concerned, it was business as usual. They were only five and four, so obviously I couldn't make us all a hot chocolate or squeeze some orange juice, sit them down and ask their thoughts on surgery.

When something important happens in my life, I forget that the whole world isn't in the know. I get so consumed with and encompassed by what I'm trying to bend my brain around that I almost think I should tell my old friend the postman my thoughts: 'Thanks for the letters. What are your thoughts on BRCA1? Would you have your breasts removed, if you had any?'

No, I didn't, really. But I did do a similarly random thing to a guy who used to work with Cian. I say 'used to', as he left of his own accord, citing a change in career.

Until now, I have never told anyone apart from Cian what I said to him.

He arrived to fit some lighting. At the time Cian was working as an interior designer, so he had lots of 'sparks', as electricians are called, working with him. 'Can I get you a cup of coffee and some of the chocolate cake I just baked?' I asked, all domestic goddess.

'Thanks, that would be lovely. Most people wouldn't give you a smack these days.' Mr Spark looked delighted.

The children were playing in the garden and out of earshot, so I guess I seized the opportunity to vent my spleen a little. I stirred my coffee slowly, my mind miles away. 'If you had a choice of having a body part cut off or dying, which would you do?'

'Wha'?' He looked at me like I was the mad one from *Misery*.

Yes, I should have made a blonde joke and left the room – but, oh no, that would've been far too easy. Me and my big mouth. I decided to educate the poor bastard on cancer genetics. '... So all I need to do now is have my breasts and ovaries removed,' I concluded. 'Would you do the same if you were in my position?'

'Erm, I've never really thought about it. I'm only nineteen, I don't have a girlfriend and there's just me and the two brothers at home. I can't say I've ever thought about women's bits in that way.' He had sweat pouring off him and looked like he'd give his last cent to be sucked out the roof by a formidable force right at that moment.

The upside of the conversation was that he could have won a Guinness World Record for the speed at which he fitted the wall lighting. There was no more idle chit-chat, no more coffee, and he didn't take his eyes off the wall until he was finished.

When Cian came home that night, I confessed I'd freaked the guy out and made him go an odd shade of green.

'I was wondering why he'd finished the job so quickly. He's usually the slowest bugger you could meet. He does a great job, but he takes forever. Maybe I'll bring a recording of you talking on the next job and he'll do the same speed trick.

'So, have you found out any more on this whole gene thing?'

'Well, I rang a specialist in the States this afternoon. His feelings on the options are a lot more black and white than over here. He basically said to have the surgery and do it quickly.'

'Easy for him to say – he's a man and he doesn't have the gene.' Cian seemed a bit annoyed.

'I don't think he was being unfeeling. He just told me what he'd say if I was his daughter,' I mused.

'How on earth did you get to talking about his children?' Cian was aghast.

'I asked him if I was his daughter, would he recommend me to have the surgery. I figure it's always good to make questions personal. It usually provokes an honest response.'

'Riiiight. I see. And I'm guessing he wasn't overjoyed to be asked that by a random stranger with an Irish leprechaun accent on the phone.'

'He answered immediately and said if his daughter had the gene he'd do the surgery himself.'

Cian was great at being interested when I woke him at three in the morning to discuss types of surgery. Just like when I was pregnant, I couldn't sleep a wink. Instead I'd sit with my laptop, logging on to all-you-need-to-know-about-surgery sites. The insomnia paid off. I had grasped enough information to make a fairly educated decision on what I was going to do.

My options were clear. I could attend a cancer clinic and be monitored, with mammograms and physical examination of the breasts. But something bothered me about the mammograms: why was the national screening programme only offered to older women? The experts told me that younger, tauter breast tissue is difficult to see through. To all intents and purposes, it was like looking into a ball of cotton wool, and so mammograms are more effective in older women. Breast cancer is also more prevalent in women over fifty. The fact that I could have regular mammograms didn't make me feel at ease. Mum had begun her continual monitoring, and as well as mammograms, she was having MRI scans of the breasts. She was happy to go that route – and although we all still hold our breath each time she goes for an examination, it's the right option for her.

With regard to the ovaries, the doctors were clear: ovarian cancer can be very difficult to detect, but they could do a transvaginal scan.

It involves the insertion of an internal probe, then pictures are taken and stored for comparison. Now in 2017 there is also a blood test available which can show doctors that ovarian cancer is either forming or already there. The patient's blood is screened and the specialist looks for the presence of a substance called CA-125. This substance is contained in all of our blood, but when certain cancers, including ovarian cancer, are growing, the level of CA-125 increases dramatically.

But back in 2005 this test wasn't an option for me, as it was only being carried out in America.

One thing I discovered about ovarian cancer freaked me out totally. It is known as the silent killer. It shows very few symptoms until it has progressed extensively. It creeps up on you, and often before you realise you have it, it's too late.

Before you throw this book across the room and run around screaming in terror, remember this. BRCA1 is rare. Only 5 per cent of cancers are hereditary. I am in a minority. Most people do not have the gene I have. The probability is that you are not going to get ovarian cancer. I am not here to scare the bejaysus out of unsuspecting people. Honestly. Let me remind you that my mum, touch wood, has never had cancer. Neither did my grandmother, and she also carried the gene. So don't feel you should jump off the nearest pier, figuring you're going to be dead soon anyway.

After the monitoring, my next option was to sit and wait. Literally to put the whole thing on the back burner and pretend it wasn't happening. But I've never liked the look of an ostrich: it has too large a body for such a small brain.

The third and final choice was the aforementioned surgery.

Two weeks had passed since I'd been told I carried the gene. I felt like one of those ticking parcels in a cartoon. I was that poor godforsaken Coyote, and Road Runner had zoomed up to me, doused me in cancer-gene dust, said, 'Meep-meep', and buggered off. I was left with wide eyes and that loud ticking, which was counting down to the explosion I was certain was going to happen.

Cian had come home late from work, tired, hungry and not in a chatty mood. But that didn't deter me. 'I want to have both my breasts removed and my ovaries gouged out,' I stated matter-of-factly.

'Is your next line going to be "Pass the salt"?' he mumbled through a mouthful of dinner.

'I've done my research, and this is the safest way of dealing with the BRCA1 gene.' I clasped my hands, propped my elbows on the table and eyeballed him.

'I've just come home from work. We found out a few days ago. I'm trying to eat. My food has mince in it. Stop talking about chopping up body parts, for the love of God!' He looked not-so-hungry now. 'Why are you staring at me like an eager puppy?'

'I think I should do it now,' I said. 'And it was two weeks ago, just for your information. Two weeks, not a few days.' I smiled in a very creepy way.

'OK, it was two weeks. Why are you looking at me with that horror-movie expression?'

'I'm ready to get this show on the road. There's no point in pissing about. I have to strike now, before it's too late.' I didn't say that I was ready to have a go myself, using some numbing sore-throat spray and my designer kitchen knives from my days as a chef.

'Well, as I said, I'm trying to eat my dinner, so you'll have to wait. Go and set up the Black & Decker Workmate and drape yourself on the floor. I'll get out the circular saw in five minutes.' His smile was all I needed. He was with me. Perhaps not that exact second, but he was on board.

For my birthday in September 2005, I got an appointment with a breast surgeon. One of my aunts, who was also looking at having the surgery, had found one in Tallaght Hospital in Dublin. Luckily, the fact that I was gene-positive meant I got an appointment very quickly. The positive part of the whole genetic conundrum was that doctors understood it was serious.

I soon realised I had two distinct fights on my hands. The first involved convincing the surgeon that I was certain I wanted the surgery carried out. The second, and by far the more frustrating, was with the hospital system. The first problem was surmountable. All that the surgeon and the breast-care nurses were aiming to do was ensure I was certain about my choice. They had the knowledge and the inclination to do the breast surgery. But they wanted me to take more time to mull over my decision.

But, as I've mentioned before, I am not a very patient person. Especially now that I wanted to become a medical patient. I remember ordering a pair of UGG boots several years ago. They had hit the headlines in fashion glossies and Elle Macpherson was in every issue sporting them. I couldn't get them locally, so I did what all women on a fashion mission do. I googled them and ordered a pair from Australia. The website promised a maximum six weeks for delivery. I waited the allotted time (amid much foot tapping). The weather became colder and my toes were bejewelled with shiny red chilblains. My patience ran out. I emailed, phoned and chased the company incessantly until my sheepskin boots arrived. I'd say they have since ceased their 'free shipping to Ireland' policy. In fact, I wouldn't be surprised if they'd commissioned the assassination of a sheep in the Wicklow hills and found a talented seamstress to custom-make my UGGs so I'd stop with the relentless emails and phone calls. (Incidentally, UGG boots are much cheaper if you buy them online – but only if you resist making long-distance phone calls to badger the suppliers!)

My eagerness and dreadful impatience raised its ugly head again when I wanted my surgery carried out.

'You're not actually sick, Emma. Take your time,' one of the nurses urged. 'Look at all the women in this corridor alone. They've been diagnosed with cancer. They have no choice but to have surgery. It's not a thing that should be taken lightly.'

I became Mrs Businesswoman about it. Right, I thought. I have to pitch for this surgery. Fine. I will. 'I'm most certainly not taking any of this lightly, and the point you've just made is exactly why I want to do this right now. I don't want to join the long queue of ladies who have cancer. I don't want to be the next in line waiting for surgery which needs to happen immediately, if not sooner. I want this done in a calm, calculated manner – before it's too late.'

'All we want is for you to be sure,' the nurses argued.

'Yes, I get that. But don't you think I've spent every waking moment – which is most of the time, I might add – mulling this over, tossing it around in my head, wondering if this is the right thing for me?'

'You're very young,' was the nurses' last-ditch attempt to stall me.

'Precisely. I'm not ready to die. I don't want to be a sitting duck and wait for cancer to strike. If I'm left for too long, I swear to God I'll manifest cancer in my breast. I have breastfed two babies. My boobs are not my fortune. I don't need them to work as a stripper or Page Three model. They've done what nature intended them to do. I'll get a new set, which will probably look a lot less saggy than these two. More than that, I'll be out of danger. I'll avoid going to the funny farm, as I slowly drive both myself and yourselves insane.'

'OK, Emma. We'll do the surgery for you.' Bingo! I was ready to go.

'So when will I come in? I can have the kids organised and all the practical stuff done in a jiffy,' I enthused.

As my surgery was elective, and being done as a preventive measure, the procedure was not seen as a priority – but, as the poor person at the UGG factory in Australia will agree, I can be very persuasive. I didn't envy my surgeon, Mr Geraghty: I chipped away and didn't let the ball drop on my campaign to make my body safer. Mr Geraghty had no illusions: he knew I was willing to have the surgery carried out by a Magimix with a brick for anaesthetic, in the public car park, if necessary. I wanted this operation done – yesterday.

My urgency reached fever pitch. The time bomb was ticking so loudly, it was threatening to go off. Tick-tock, tick-tock. I needed to defuse it before it could even attempt to wipe me out.

We all see the TV news, with images of people on trolleys in corridors, the elderly and gravely ill waiting to be seen. I knew the public hospital system was in rag order. But until it landed on my lap and affected me personally, it hadn't been real.

In January 2006, nearly six months after I'd been diagnosed with BRCA1, the surgical team and I were ready to go. I spoke to the oncology nurses in Tallaght at length. I took on board that, although he would do his best, Mr Geraghty might not be able to save my nipples. I knew my reconstruction would be gradual. After removing the breast tissue, Mr Geraghty would place expanding bags behind the muscles on my chest wall. Week after week, I would go in to have saline injected into them. The bags would create a pocket for the breast implants to live in. It would be a minimum of eight months later that I could have the implants put in place.

I knew the road ahead would be long and difficult. I was fully aware that it wasn't going to be easy. But that was fine. I was taking control. I was leading the way. I was changing my destiny. Instead of being a sitting target, and quivering in my boots, I was standing up and shouting, 'NO. I am not going to allow this genetic predisposition to destroy me.'

Chapter 6

Are We There Yet?

Are we there yet? Are we there yet? Is the answer just around the next corner? Will I know in five more minutes? Will I? Huh? Huh? Ah, yes – surgery part one is abreast.

I have a special talent for wearing people down. I have come to the slightly surprised realisation that I have quite a lot in common with Mrs Doyle from *Father Ted*. She was on a mission to get the world to drink tea. She had a goal in life and, in fairness to her, she put her heart and soul into achieving it. I understood her crusade. In a similar way, in spite of the lagging hospital system, I managed to get a fixed date – or so I thought.

I was to go in on Sunday, 15 January 2006. I would spend the night (or have 'one sleep', as Kim put it) and the surgery was scheduled for Monday, 16 January.

Once that was settled in my head, a whole new nest of nuisances came to light. Who was going to clean the toilets while I was incapacitated? I am the only person in our house who knows how to change a toilet roll. Cian and the children are capable in many ways, but none of them seems to know how to remove the empty cardboard tube and replace it with a new roll.

Who would wash the clothes? The system up until then involved dumping all the dirty stuff on the floor. The washing-machine elf would scuttle in, while everyone was at school and work, wash, dry and iron the stuff, then put it away.

Who was going to pick the bits of crisps and popcorn out of the sofa? Who would know where Sacha's Wii controller was? Who would find the missing chair so all the Sylvanians could sit for dinner?

Mum and Dad offered to help. Just before Kim was born in 2001, we had built a house in my parents' garden. What used to be an orchard is now our home. Although the apple and pear trees were nearly a century old, and had long since stopped bearing fruit, I did feel mean uprooting them and pouring foundations over their previous habitat. Luckily we have never been haunted by human-sized angry Cox's Orange Pippins, vowing to take revenge for our having destroyed their cousins.

Cian's parents, Orlaith and Seán, were the same in offering their help. But all of them work. All of them have lives. I was in the fortunate position of being able to afford an au pair. I had enough time to find a girl who could speak enough English, and wield an iron and a hoover with a sunny disposition.

Jane was our shining light. From Slovakia, she had already spent enough time in Ireland to make friends. At any moment when we didn't need her, she was gone, looking for pints to drink and boys to bat her eyes at. Perfect. I couldn't have coped with another person to worry about and I didn't have to. She was a joy to live with and had the constitution of an ox.

The preparations *chez nous* were carried out with military precision. I made lasagne, stews and pies for the freezer. The whole family had a copy of the children's rota, which I'd typed and printed and gone through with everyone *ad nauseam*. (It's beside the point that all the stuff was still in the same position in the freezer two months later.) Sacha and Kim told me in wide-eyed delight that Jane made the best breakfast in the world. It involved marshmallows and chocolate spread, so it was easy to understand why.

I had been told by the hospital to phone just after lunch to confirm my bed. Just before Cian and I were due to set off for Tallaght, I made the quick call.

'Yes, Emma Hannigan. I see your name on the list here. I'm sorry, there's no bed available today. You'll have to phone through to the breast-care unit tomorrow and they should be able to help you with rescheduling,' the receptionist shrilled.

'What do you mean? That's it? My surgery's cancelled – there's no information and no explanation? Go away?' My eyes were welling, my hands were shaking and I honestly thought I was going to collapse.

'I don't have any further information at this desk. Sorry about that.'

That was, hand on heart, the most devastating time of my entire journey. My decision to have the genetic test done – easy. My decision to have the radical surgery – easy. To have my surgery cancelled with no warning and absolutely no comeback – sheer torture.

I threw the cordless phone on the bed and locked myself in the bathroom. Sitting on the toilet lid, I could hear Jane helping the children into coats. The plan had been to take them for burgers and chips while Cian drove me to the hospital. It sounds crazy, but I couldn't go down the stairs and tell them it wasn't happening. I thought of Cian, my parents, his parents, all our friends.

'Emma?' Cian knocked on the bathroom door.

'I'll be out in a minute.' The tears choked me.

'You'll be OK. It's nearly over. I'll stay as long as you like in the hospital this evening.'

'It's cancelled. They're not doing it.' I opened the door to face him.

'What?' The silence was deafening. We were flummoxed. We were also powerless.

'But they can't do that to you.' Cian was furious.

'They can and they have. There's fuck-all we can do about it.'

Cian made another call to the hospital and, despite ranting and raving, got no joy. There was nobody available to speak to us: none of the medical team whom I'd been dealing with were there on a Sunday.

Despite several phone calls, it was three days before I even managed to speak to anyone of relevance. They were all very sorry, they regretted having had to cancel the surgery, but it was out of their hands. Accident & Emergency was inundated: all the surgical beds had been allotted. Full stop.

'But have you any idea of the psychological impact these cancellations have on patients?' I argued.

'We all know it's really hard, but the system is so blocked and the public hospitals are so overstretched that this kind of thing happens all the time.' The nurse sighed. 'If it helps at all, we have to work with this kind of thing happening to our patients week after week. It's horrendous from our point of view too. None of us wants to see patients distressed. That's not what we signed up for when we entered the medical profession.'

I knew it wasn't personal. I knew it wasn't the nurses' or the doctors' fault, but at the end of the day the person suffering most in that situation was me. Unfortunately I am not alone. So many others have been on news programmes since then, trying to get someone to listen to the plight of patients on waiting lists and hospital trolleys. I hope with all my heart the system changes for the better – and fast.

Chapter 7

Anyone for Swapsies?

Does anyone remember Multi-Coloured Swap Shop *in the eighties? Where you could ring and offer unwanted toys for stuff your parents wouldn't let you have? I like the finer things in life. So I'm willing to exchange my goose-down duvet for a rubber sheet. Or a fine glass of Bordeaux for a saline drip.*

Perhaps I hadn't had enough upset, so some bad fairy with a grudge decided to push me a little further. I was due to have the operation on 13 February 2006 – but guess what? Oh, yes. The system got in the way again. I was majorly upset but, as Rod Stewart wisely pointed out, the first cut is in fact the deepest. By that point I think I'd almost reached deflation stage. I wanted to fight my corner, but it was futile. I was up against the enormous beast that was crushing so many patients. The fact that I was a private patient with full medical insurance made no difference to my outcome.

Eventually, emotionally exhausted, I got a bed. It was 26 February 2006, almost six weeks after the original surgery date. By that time I should have been well on my way to recovery. I have never been so pleased to lie on a crunchy-sounding bed, fitted with a rubber sheet, waiting to be taken to a chilled room and chopped up by a man in a mask with a very sharp knife. The moment had arrived. Finally the danger was going to be removed. Only 'one more sleep' as a person with real breast tissue. I looked at my watch. Nine o'clock in the evening. The surgery was going to take eight hours. Removing entire breasts took much longer than putting in implants. For all the world, I needed to be filleted. There was a whole new meaning to 'chicken fillets' in bras in my head!

By nine o'clock the following night, I would be through the operation. I contemplated my breasts. How did I feel about them finally going? I was truly excited. I was certain I was never going to regret what I was doing. I would never have a moment of panic and think, 'Quick, scoop it all out of the bin and give it back.' I was losing some breast tissue. I was gaining life.

At that point the world of surgery was foreign to me, so the hordes of people shuffling around in Crocs, green scrubs uniforms and speaking in muffled tones through masks were fascinating. The surgical area of the hospital was like a huge swimming pool: it was all sea-green tiles, from walls to floors. Everything looked sterile and clean.

'Is it made like this so you can power-hose all the blood off the walls and floors easily?' I asked the nurse.

'I've never really thought about the decor but, yes, it needs to be easy to keep clean.' She smiled as she asked me to move from the wheelchair I'd been transported in.

The trolley-style bed I clambered onto was like the one at the beautician's, except it had a big blue cooler-bag mat on it. You know those things you put in your insulated picnic bag to keep stuff cold? Imagine gluing a load of them together: you have a surgical mat.

'I'll just get you another pillow and a blanket to make you more comfortable.' She patted my arm kindly. I was going to tell her that comfy was about as far from this situation as it was possible to be, but I didn't want to sound rude.

The softness of the pillow and blue waffle blanket did indeed help matters. I could close my eyes and pretend I was waiting for a leg wax rather than having my breasts removed.

'I'm going to wheel the bed into the pre-op room now. Hold on tight, Emma.'

I found myself in a rectangular room, not much bigger than a broom cupboard, with shelves on either side containing clear plastic packages of needles, tubes and other medical paraphernalia.

'Hi, Emma, I'm going to be making sure you don't feel anything or wake up.' The anaesthetist appeared, like Mr Benn, from behind my head. The entire situation was surreal. I should probably have been freaking out, shaking and bursting into tears, but instead I just felt my heart beating faster – no doubt I was nervous, but I wasn't terrified. I had yearned for this moment for so many weeks that it was almost on a par with Christmas morning when I was a child. Adrenalin must've taken over and stopped me having a meltdown.

The anaesthetist will forever remain up there with Switzerland's finest chocolate. He was a smiley sort of chap – well, his eyes were crinkly and friendly, but his mouth and the rest of his face were obscured by his mask. He also had a tendency to shout, which is very beneficial. Have you ever tried to hear what someone is saying when you can't see their mouth? It's not that easy. Try it. So, this guy was a bit on the loud side, and unquenchably cheerful.

'How's it going?' (Crinkly eyes.)

'I've been better, but I've also been worse. I'm so relieved to finally be here,' I said.

'Jaysus, rather you than me. You're very brave. Don't think I could do it.' He shook his head. No crinkly eyes this time, but raised eyebrows instead.

'Well, I'd say it would be difficult enough to remove your breasts. From what I can see through your scrubs, you don't have much in the way of man-boobs going on there.' He was a greyhound figure of a man.

The crinkles were back. 'What'll we talk about? I've to hold you here for ten minutes, which can seem like a decade in your position. Would you like some magic juice to relax you for starters?' he offered.

'Love some. Bring it on.' I smiled. If I'd been at the Ritz-Carlton, I wouldn't have felt as pampered. I'm not a person who ever took many pills and potions, but right then, I would've gladly taken heroin had they offered it to me. It was just like that feeling on the morning of your wedding, or as you walk into a room at a big function, when a waiter appears with a tray of wine or champagne. Most of us dive into a glass of Dutch courage, knowing it will help to bolster us up. This was just the same, and the man with the drugs was my very best friend.

The magic juice turned out to be some marvellous fuzzy stuff, which he injected into the bit of Lego in my hand. It was a bit stingy on the veins for a couple of seconds but, oh, so worth the pain. Why this stuff isn't given to all people over the age of one on a regular basis is beyond me. Perhaps it might cause liver damage or kidney failure if used too often but, take it from me, we'd all die ecstatic. There would be very few problems left in the world.

We chatted about Crème de la Mer face cream and Jimmy Choo shoes. Oh, OK, I did all the garbled talking and poor Crinkly Eyes nodded kindly and patted my arm simultaneously.

I was devastated when the surgical team called me in. I'd say Crinkly Eyes was ready to mix the dose vets use to put animals out of their misery. God bless him, he waved and wished me well, and I waved back so vigorously I nearly fell off the trolley.

My first thought when I woke up after the operation was, 'Thank God I wasn't dreaming: it's finally happened.' As the porter was wheeling me back to the ward, Cian walked towards me. 'She's totally out of it,' the porter said to him, in a thick Dublin accent.

My eyes didn't have the power to open, but I was wide awake on the inside. Under the veil of drugs I was fully aware. I've heard of cases where patients have been in a coma, often for a long time. They can hear and remember everything that's going on around them, but they can't communicate. This was exactly the same.

Round one to me. I had survived the surgery. Everything after that would fall into place. I'd had this dreadful fear that I was going to be one of those patients who reacted adversely to anaesthetic and croaked it on the operating table. Imagine what a pisser that would have been. I could see the headlines: 'Bray woman dies trying to save own life'. The fact that I looked like a pile of tubes with eyes was immaterial.

I was able to keep the skin over where my breasts had been and, amazingly, Dr Geraghty had managed to save both nipples, so I still looked 'normal'. Well, if the truth be told, none of it actually looked 'normal' for quite a while. But I knew I was on the way there. The incisions were made at the side of my breast, just under my armpits and all the tissue had been removed. I had been filleted beautifully.

So, how did I feel? Any regrets?

Absolutely none. I felt nothing but relief and a wonderful sense of achievement. The surgery had taken almost nine hours, but the team were all delighted with the results. Just to give you a little visual: I was flat-chested, with drains, a drip and little bags to collect the fluid that drained off the operated-on area. For the day after the operation I couldn't move much. But the nurses soon had me up and about. Well, I did a kind of shuffling stoop while I dragged the drip and drains around. I can't say I looked overly attractive – I had the complexion of a three-week-old corpse, and I hadn't washed my hair for three days, so it was now sporting the oil-slick-on-a-muddy-field look.

Under normal circumstances I won't even go outside without make-up on. I'm just not comfortable sporting the 'natural look'. I have very pale skin, pale eyes and pale hair. So, unaided by the marvels of make-up, I look and feel like death warmed up. But as I moved around the hospital like a clockwork dolly, with manky hair, no make-up and no boobs, did I care? Hand on heart – no.

I love my clothes and accessories just as much as the next girl, but during that time, I was in survival mode. All things in life are relative. At that stage, the main objective was recovery. Everything else was immaterial. I realised that I was able to put things in perspective. The main thing was that I would hopefully have plenty of time in the future to put on my face, wash my hair, wear flattering clothes and look the best I could.

My arms were a bit glued to my sides, turfing my usual skin routine out the window, so I was developing a nice teenage-acne look. Why is it that at times of heightened distress or worry your skin erupts? When you're feeling like poo, spots or really sore boils always appear. I understand it's because your immune system is low, yadda, yadda, but it's dreadfully unfair, isn't it? How many people do we all know who woke up on the morning before their wedding with a dose of cold sores that made the Elephant Man look like a supermodel? Cruel.

The nurses had told me that, even though I was stiff and sore, the worst thing I could do was lie there and not move. 'A bit of pain at this stage will really stand to you. It will keep everything from going into spasm,' one of the chatty nurses had advised.

So I took her literally and made sure to haul myself out of bed as often as I could bear. It was all a bit of a military operation. I needed help to get up because of the drip and drains, but once I was on my feet, I could do my own rusty version of the Moonwalk in pink slippers. Each time I got up I tried to go a little further than the time before. By day three I was clearing the end of the ward and even managing to make it out the door towards the lift.

I was doing my geriatric-with-advanced-polio shuffle up the corridor, dragging my drip and drains, when the lift door pinged open. My neck was too stiff, and I was too terrified of twisting my body to look around.

'Dear God, you're lucky you're married. The state of you!'

'Shut up, I can't laugh or my drains will fall off.' I shook with giggles as Cian came up behind me.

I am not the type of person who reacts well to pity. Cian knew if he'd come in with watery eyes, tried to hug me and tell me that I was doing great, I would have mustered all my strength to strangle him with my tubes. He is my perfect balance: he knows when to step back and when to be there. When I was really sick and in pain, he took the piss out of me. Even if I was contemplating suicide, he would somehow make me smile. Laughter truly is the best medicine.

I had taken my first step in the right direction. Little by little, I was making my body as hostile as I could to cancer. The major surgery was over. I had started the biggest journey of my life. The sense of personal achievement was immense.

Chapter 8

Life on the Inside

Being somewhat institutionalised is oddly liberating. Mealtimes, drug times and bedtimes are all decided for you. No brainer. It's a bit like a holiday camp with white coats ...

I can't say I ever felt I'd missed out by not attending a boarding school. I'd always loved and appreciated the privilege of my own bedroom at home, so I was mildly nervous of life on the inside – in the hospital, that is.

It's an odd one. You're obviously all there because you have to be, for either surgery or treatment, and, due to the forced-room-mate situation, there's an atmosphere of mutual respect, which is nice.

I stayed in hospital for a week after the surgery. I found the dynamics of the place fascinating. The ward was like a soap opera. Perhaps because none of us was looking hot, it was like all the regular rules no longer applied. In many ways it was a bit like being back in school again. By that I mean we were all in uniform – pyjamas. No make-up, jewellery or toys were allowed. We all had to do what Teacher (the nurses) said. The only form of competition was in the number of bouquets we received and who had the most red lemonade on their locker.

There was a bit of war-victim rivalry, but not in a nasty way. Any new patient who arrived on the ward would be allowed to settle before one of us asked: 'So, what are you in for?'

There was a little mother-hen lady in the bed beside the window. She was in for a gall-bladder removal and had caught an infection.

She had been there longest and had appointed herself head girl. She did the smiling and nodding at newbies. She had a deft talent for sucking all sorts of information out of people. Even the ones who, like me, tried to keep their curtains shut as far as possible. Oh, no, there was no escape. I soon realised that it was easier to come clean and tell the audience why I was there.

Mother-hen cleverly volunteered her entire life story, from conception to the current day, all in one breath. She was a heavy smoker, so she had to keep dragging her drip outside to the smoking area, which to me was an awful lot of hassle. But the fags obviously weren't affecting her lung capacity. I'm convinced she had some kind of contraption inserted in the back of her head that breathed for her while she spoke. It was astonishing how many words she could squeeze into each deep breath. Once she'd finished telling the latest newbie and all the other inmates (again) why she was there, she would leave an expectant pause. Of course, you'd feel obliged to tell her all your private details.

There was a certain freedom in the ward. We were all from different parts of the country and, unless Mrs Gall Bladder was planning a reunion dinner, none of us had any intention of ever seeing each other again. So it was fine to tell random strangers that you'd just had your breasts lopped off, spleen removed or womb sucked out.

The other reason Herself was allowed be mother-hen was her ability to go shopping. I wasn't mobile enough due to my drip and drains. Others were also hooked up to various contraptions, so we were stuck. Herself could take orders and hobble to the lobby. The shop was just beside the smoking hut too: not only would she come back with the stuff we wanted, but a whole new repertoire of tales from the other smokers. If we thought we were impressive in our ward, we were only Montessori level compared with the hardened smokers' class. Herself had even met a man who'd had his leg amputated. I'm not usually the type of person who would relish a conversation about circulation being cut off and toes dropping into wellies and eventual amputation. But when you're stuck in a room with five others 24/7, you'll listen to anything. It's a bit like that reality TV show when the celebrities are in the jungle. After the initial shock at their surroundings, they all loll around having utterly mindless conversations about their cleaning ladies selling their under-pants on eBay.

There were plenty of visitors, but as it was a public hospital, the times were strictly monitored. Televisions were big business: they were only available to hire. When the TV guy came around, Mother-hen took charge of bargaining with him. She was like a Moore Street trader when it came to money changing hands. We all chipped in to hire the television for the week. It was a fairly pointless exercise, as it was too small to watch and the noise of the clattering trolleys made it impossible to hear. If the truth be known, it just added a dull mumble to the railway-station din. But I wasn't about to tell Herself that we didn't need it.

Newspapers were another communal effort. Woe betide the rebel who would hobble to the shop and purchase a newspaper without consulting Herself first. No edition could be bought twice, and the minute you were finished reading, you had to offer it up for the next person. Glossy magazines were frowned upon, and I had to say that all of mine were presents – and most of them were, but they were forbidden because you could feed a family in Africa for a week for the price of one. Weeklies were allowed though, especially the ones about diets.

I was the only non-obese inmate on my ward. But I was still allowed to join in with the starve-yourself chat. The hospital food was beyond description. All of it managed to smell like nursing home; most of it resembled the contents of a baby's nappy. So we had a lot of picnics. Most of them involved sandwiches from the shop, garnished with bags of crisps and bars of chocolate. There were endless boxes of chocolates brought by well-wishers, which the ladies (including myself) would post into their beaks on a constant basis.

'I eat very little,' Mother-hen used to muse, between mouthfuls of Cherry Bakewell, mixed with mini-Snickers, all washed down with a bucket of red lemonade. 'So it's not my fault that I'm well padded.'

'My family are all overweight, so I'm never going to be thin,' agreed another inmate.

'Do you know what really bothers me?' Mrs Second-from-the-left was flushed with emotion. 'In fact, "bother" is the wrong word. It pisses me off, excuse my French.' She shook her head.

'What, love?' Mother-hen leaned forwards.

'That some gobshite went and changed the name of a Marathon to a Snickers. It put me right off them. It sounds too much like "knickers". Can't eat them any more.'

'I know what you mean,' Mother-hen agreed. 'So what are ya in for then, love?'

Nicely executed, I thought, with a smile.

Mrs Second-from-the-left was from the flats in inner-city Dublin and had her own marvellous way of expressing herself. 'I'm here to have me gearbox hoovered out (otherwise commonly known as a hysterectomy),' she'd announced, totally unabashed.

'Why are you in here, love?' All eyes turned to me. Mother-hen sat up straight. 'Wait till you hear this. Fantastic she is, I'd be devastated if I'd been mutilated the way this one has.'

I laughed and told Mrs Newbie why I was there. Needless to say, she sat agog and told me she couldn't face her pint of lemonade after I'd filled her in.

I never saw the surgery as mutilation. Nor did I feel like less of a woman after the operation. My boobs had done their job with the kids and it was time for them to go.

I vividly remember Mr Geraghty popping his head around the curtains on the morning after the op. 'Are we still friends?' he asked tentatively.

God love him, he had spent the night worrying that I might have changed my mind. That I would tell him to run after the bin lorry, scoop all the breast tissue out and shove it back in.

I guess, even to a breast surgeon, what I'd had done appeared radical. But he didn't have the image of my Aunt Helen lying with a posy of lily-of-the-valley in her clasped hands. I did. Tubes and scars may not be pretty, but I knew that time would heal all of that. Now I had time. The reason I had opted for the double mastectomy was so clear in my head. I had changed my destiny and prolonged my life. I was using the knowledge that genetic testing had provided and I was pre-empting the worst-case scenario. I was fighting the good fight, and it felt so good.

Slowly but surely I got better. The drains were pulled out. The drip came down. The pain medication switched to an oral version. I was good to go. I was beyond excited about my discharge, but a tiny part of me would miss the reports from the smokers' hut and the picnics.

Chapter 9

The Amazing Inflatable Woman

Pimp My Breasts. Well, pump them to be exact. I'm the amazing inflatable woman!

By the end of March 2006, I was allowed to begin having my breast expanders filled. This involved going to the day-surgery area of the hospital and having saline injected into them. Because the skin and muscle have to expand slowly, I had to go in every two weeks for a top-up. By the end of April, the correct amount of saline had been put into the bags. I had to wait a further six months before the muscle pocket would be ready to take a silicone implant.

By now, I was used to the antiseptic smell of the hospital. I no longer noticed the stark corridors or the echoing air of sickness. It was almost like a home from home.

The fun part about all this was that I could suddenly wear all sorts of tops and dresses that were previously out of bounds to a mother who'd breast-fed two babies. A lot of women look at halter-neck backless dresses with envy, knowing that they no longer have the collagen, elastin, muscle tone or youth to appear in public in said garments for fear of giving themselves or an unsuspecting passer-by a black eye. The biggest advantage of my newly pumped-up breasts was that they didn't require a bra.

'Look!' I took off my cardigan in a coffee shop and showed my astonished friends my new shape. Turning around with plenty of eyebrow-raising, I revealed the fact that my back wasn't punctuated with an ugly bra strap.

'Oh, my God, they stay up on their own!' one of the girls exclaimed.

'Certainly do! Now I'll be able to buy all the backless gowns in sales that nobody else could bear to spend money on, knowing they'd have to spend the same amount of money again on expensive under-wear!'

By the end of May 2006 I felt ready to start along the road to ovary removal. I wanted to have all my surgery completed within a year. Perhaps it was just my way of putting the whole process in perspective: if I knew it wasn't going to go on forever, it would be easier to cope with. Determined to keep to my schedule, I arranged for Cian and me to meet the gynaecological surgeon. He outlined what the operation would entail. Using keyhole surgery, they would make a small incision in my abdomen and also access my insides via my belly button.

When I heard that, my cringeometer went into overdrive. I am not remotely squeamish but I don't do belly buttons. I think they're creepy and look like little portholes to the parts of your body that nobody needs to think about. Yuck.

'I need to remove both Fallopian tubes also, as they can harbour cells from the ovaries.'

'Fine by me,' I confirmed.

'The operation should only take around forty minutes and you shouldn't be too uncomfortable afterwards.'

The surgeon was a man. Need I say more? He'd never had a baby or considered having his ovaries and Fallopian tubes removed – oh, wait, he didn't have any, did he? So, it was fine for him to make a comment like that.

'You have to come in and see a psychologist, just so we have it on record that you both fully understand your fertility will be no more after this operation.'

I wanted to point out that I wasn't stupid, so I was well aware that my fertile days might just be over once my ovaries and Fallopian tubes were removed, but seeing as this man was going to be wielding a very sharp knife in my presence while I was unconscious, I thought it might be wise not to piss him off.

We were lucky to get an appointment on 23 June 2006 for our psychological assessment.

'So do you reckon they'll pronounce us clinically insane and have the children put into care?' I quipped, as Cian and I entered the hospital.

'Just so long as you don't rock violently and make repeated high-pitched noises, you should be OK.'

We followed the signs to the area I'd been instructed to go to.

'You'd want to be sick to come in here.' Cian stood with his arms folded beside the line of plastic bucket seats. 'Why are the chairs nailed to the floor in a row? Nobody in their right mind would even think of nicking them.'

'Why don't you sit down and stop blocking up the hallway with the I'm-a-bouncer pose?' I smiled.

'No, thanks, I'm fine here.' He paced uncomfortably, like a caged animal. I watched as he peered around his surroundings unhappily. 'Not the nicest place on the planet, is it?' he commented.

'I suppose not. I don't really notice any more. I've become so used to being here that it doesn't really bother me now.'

I was glad we weren't kept waiting that day. It was one thing for me to have to sit for hours in the corridor, but I didn't want to inflict that on Cian. He was being so supportive, backing me up emotionally and practically, and I didn't want to add hours of point-less waiting to the list of things he had to endure.

To me, my ovaries were in the same boat as my breasts. They had performed like Formula One parts in their day. Cian and I were very lucky to have had no bother in conceiving, and we had decided well before we'd even heard of BRCA1 that our family was complete. With Sacha and Kim in school, I had just got to the light at the end of the baby-minding tunnel. I'd bought a handbag that was so small it didn't dislocate my shoulder when I picked it up. I'd changed the car seats from the ones that require a month's training at NASA to operate in favour of the little booster ones. We'd had all the food-encrusted carpets at home scrapped and replaced them with shiny wooden floors and rugs. I'd even joined a Pilates class and managed to turn up at it several times in a row. So, for us, the decision was an easy one.

All the same, there were steps we had to take to convince the hospital of our certainty. Everyone needed to know that we were happy to end our fertile days as a couple.

The psychologist who met us that day in June began by apologising.

'Sorry we're so cramped in here.' The room was like a broom closet. 'Sorry it's me you're attending, but this is kind of an odd situation.'

'Why? What's wrong with you?' Cian eyeballed her suspiciously.

'Nothing – it's just that I'm actually a child psychologist. But nobody else has come looking to make this decision yet, and while they put the relevant person in place, I'm standing in.' I've no doubt she was wonderful with children. She looked about twelve and struck me as one of those adults who are much happier in the company of toddlers than they are with grown-ups.

Her usual props, which consisted of a Barney glove puppet and flash cards, weren't that useful for us. I could see her itching to find a tool of some sort to help with our session. 'I don't suppose we need to do role-play for this one?' It could have been my paranoia, but I could've sworn she would have happily put her hand up the dinosaur's bottom if we'd encouraged it even slightly.

Luckily for all concerned, we were certain of what we wanted to do.

'I am going to ask you both in turn. Would you like to have another baby before you go ahead with this surgery?' The psychologist looked to me first. 'You're both still young. You've had the bilateral mastectomy, which has already reduced your risks.' Now she was unabashedly reading from an A4 sheet. 'You have time to have more children now, if that's what you both want.'

Indeed, had I wanted to hold off for a while, the fact that I had removed my breast tissue meant my odds of getting cancer were much lower than the original 85 per cent. With the BRCA1 gene, the ovaries and breast tissue were the two influencing factors for danger. Because I had removed one element, I had already made myself safer.

There was a brief silence. Expectation hung in the air. Without making eye contact with Cian, I answered from the bottom of my heart. 'Thanks for trying to sound convincing when you said we were young. I'm sure you really think we're both ready for puréed food and guided bus tours to Llandudno. But I am finished. As far as I'm concerned, the baby shop is shut. The thought of having to get up every two hours at night fills me with suicidal tendencies.' The therapist nodded gravely.

'Oh, thank Christ.' Cian exhaled and a smile formed on his previously stricken face.

Before you think for even one second that either of us was being flippant or callous, reconsider. Children are, without a shadow of a doubt, the most amazing thing that ever happened to us. Although the baby stage is relentless, with 24/7 wiping of orifices and disposing of soiled, soggy articles, I would never hesitate to recommend it. But I have to admit to basking in the fact that I had reached the stage where I could wear things like white jeans and not have a chocolate handprint on them a whole hour later. I could meet a friend for coffee (yes, I am still an addict) and nobody would scream or try to run out the door or pour the milk into the sugar bowl.

However, I do think there could be a book in which people tell the truth about parenting. No book I've ever read told me that you sleep with one eye open forever after you've given birth, that you suddenly become the proud owner of an in-built microchip which causes you to worry about every step and breath your child takes, not to mention anticipating all sorts of awfulness that might just happen in the future – all at four in the morning.

When Kim was still being weighed in the delivery room, Cian was already pacing up and down, telling the team of midwives how he was going to have to go clubbing with her and interview all her future boyfriends in the basement with a baseball bat.

But they are the negative aspects. The joy and love and sheer enjoyment that our children have bestowed upon us are magical. They have enriched Cian and me in more ways than we will ever be able to appreciate. They are one of the main reasons we both have for living.

But we were happy with what we'd got. One of each flavour: a boy and a girl. Both healthy and happy. We simply felt complete.

'But what if your marriage were to break down? Emma, you might like to have a baby with your new partner.' The psychologist was playing devil's advocate.

'No. The new partner would need to have children from a previous relationship if he wanted to be a daddy,' I answered.

'Or else he could just dote on ours. Would he like to pay the school fees, do you reckon?' Cian joked. We were both giggling and poking each other. The psychologist wasn't laughing. She was sitting poker-faced, waiting for a proper answer.

'I don't want to have any more children, not with Cian or any potential hypothetical non-existent partner in the future.' I kept a straight face and didn't look at Cian.

'Me too.' He nodded, smirking.

'Well, you can go and find a young one and she can have your babies, if you want,' I jibed.

'Why are you allowed to go off with someone and not have babies, and I have to be with a teenage baby machine?' He smiled.

A soft cough from the psychologist silenced us. We were never allowed to see the report she filed, but I would hazard a guess that she recommended removal of both ovaries with immediate effect, while also asking to be sterilised herself. I was phoned the following morning and given a date just over ten days later − 4 July − for my surgery.

'I'd say she wrote in black indelible pen, in block capitals: "Remove her ovaries, give him a vasectomy and put them in separate cells in the nuthouse."' Cian laughed.

I had to agree it seemed like too much of a coincidence that I was suddenly being called for surgery without having to wait for months. 'They'll probably cancel it twice, so we could potentially have one or two babies by the time they actually take me in,' I mused.

Part two of my surgery was imminent. I was heading for the next chapter of my story. In the same way as before, I was filled with determination sprinkled with trepidation. I wasn't nervous. It was far too positive for that. I didn't view this operation as a bad thing. It was a great thing. It was going to help me survive!

Chapter 10

Ovaries, Au Revoir

*It's been nice knowing you: you've served me well and done a
fine job producing two perfect children, but your time is up …*

The school year ended at the beginning of June 2006, so we were
looking at three months of free time with no need to haul the
children out of bed and rush them out the door. Sicily beckoned. I
was excited about the idea of two weeks away from hospitals, school,
work and the humdrum routine of everyday life. It was going to be
like paradise for the four of us. We could spend some quiet time in
the sunshine and take stock of everything. I knew my ovary surgery
was looming so 'headspace' was exactly what the doctor ordered.

In theory it was fantastic. In reality, Sacha vomited repeatedly on
the transfer from the airport, as we travelled in an overcrowded
non-air-conditioned bus at a speed Michael Schumacher would've
been proud of along a road that looked like it was framing the edge
of the earth. Sheer drops: it was blood-curdling, a journey I'd say
the devil has marked as a favourite in his personal satellite navigation
system.

We arrived alive and just about in one piece, with a green-tinged
miserable son and a cranky daughter, to discover we'd landed ourselves
in a modern-day version of a Butlin's holiday camp. The reason we'd
chosen that particular resort was because it boasted a vast range of
activities, from circus-style training to skateboarding. What they had
failed to mention was that the rooms were just one step up from
camping in the luxury stakes. Of course, our children were the only

61

ones in the whole complex to take one look at the kids' club and do open-mouthed howling, followed by full-on refusal to leave my side.

Cian made tons of friends and became obsessed with everything from basketball to rollerblading. Sacha and Kim spent the entire time in the swimming pool. I spent the two weeks wrapping them in towels and trooping them from one buffet to the next. Although I loved the quality-time concept and we created lots of lovely memories (honestly), hand-washing children's clothes in a cracked sink and anticipating the return bus journey along the highway to hell was not the happiest time of my life. If the truth be known, I was never so happy to touch down in Dublin airport.

Shortly after our holiday I was back into the swing of all things surgical.

When 4 July 2006 dawned, my cousins in the States were preparing to have the barbecue of the year, and I was donning a hospital robe, then walking down the stairs to the surgery department. I kept thinking it was all too good to be true. I only believed the surgery was finally going ahead when I met the anaesthetist and he injected the magic fuzzy juice into my vein.

Thankfully, the surgery went according to plan. Both ovaries and Fallopian tubes were removed successfully. After my mastectomy I had suffered an adverse reaction to morphine, with itchy skin, hallucinations and shaking, and it hadn't killed the pain. Now the pain specialist had to find a balance with other drugs. As a result, I was kept in Recovery for four hours. An operation that was meant to be quick seemed to go on for a very long time.

Unfortunately there was a breakdown in communication with the ward. I had kissed Cian goodbye at around eleven that morning. By the time I arrived back up from Recovery at five thirty that evening, Cian had booked the plot and had the children picking out hymns for the funeral mass. I was groggy and in dreadful pain. My abdomen felt like it had been cleaned out with an apple corer. As Cian did his Sudoku puzzle, I dozed in and out of reality.

What felt like ten seconds later, the nurse on duty came over and told me to get out of the bed and get ready to go home.

'She's just come back from Recovery.' Cian looked perplexed.

'This is a day ward and it closes at six. We're all going home in ten minutes, so you have to leave.'

To say that Cian hit the roof is putting it mildly. He ushered the nurse to the end of the ward and stood with her out of my earshot, but I could see him through the double-glazed window. His head took on a kind of beetroot appearance, as his nostrils flared to twelve times their normal size. He did pointing and snappy arm-folding, followed by hands-on-hips. 'Ha-ha' type noises filtered towards me. But I knew he wasn't laughing.

In fact, I was seriously fearful that he was going to march off like a man possessed and find some suitable implement, anything ranging from a biro to the leg of a chair, to perform similar surgery on the staff to what I'd just endured.

Himself and the staff nurse came back in to look at me.

'If you were lying there with your insides carved out, doped to the eyeballs and writhing in pain, would you relish the thought of getting dressed and going on an adventure down the M50 motorway?'

Cian pointed at me. I felt slightly under pressure to look very stricken, suddenly wondering if I should allow my tongue to hang out my mouth or do some sort of animal moan. The fact of the matter was that I didn't have the energy to do either, so I just lay there and hoped I looked as shite as I felt.

There was mumbling and hushed talk from the nurse, with plenty of blinking and frozen smiles.

Cian was less friendly and much louder. 'I am not interested in whether or not you think it's a day ward. Find another place to put that bed. It's on wheels – it's not rocket science. Bring it to where there are nurses on duty. In fact, you tell me where to go and I'll do it myself.'

I was so groggy and sore, I had to have a quick bit of shut-eye. I hoped that if I gave in to the druggy stupor for a short while, the arm-waving and arguing might be over.

But it was futile. Guess what? There were no beds available in the hospital. My only option would be to go on a trolley in A & E and wait my turn. As it was, there were allegedly eight people in the corridor who were ahead of me in the line for beds.

'So, you're telling me that in this entire place' – Cian was now doing sweeping windmill gestures, with rather crazy eye-popping stares thrown in – 'You expect me to really believe that there is not a broom cupboard or patch of space to wheel that bed and have a nurse monitor her?'

'Yes, I am.'

'Fantastic. Just brilliant.' Cian had finished waving. His voice was barely audible. He was rubbing his face vigorously with his hands.

I didn't know what to do. I hated putting him through the stress. I didn't want to be the cause of all this trouble. But if I stayed there, I would probably have to stand like a drunk horse in A & E where the only thing on offer that night was MRSA. Understandably, I decided to go home.

Cian went to find a wheelchair and a porter to help manoeuvre me. I couldn't bend over to dress myself so we stuffed my clothes into the overnight bag. Cian put on my shoes and socks and I draped my coat over my shoulders. By the time I reached the front door of the hospital, the motion of the wheelchair was making me nauseous. I felt like I'd spent four hours on the waltzers, while drinking a bottle of crème de menthe. For future reference, a general anaesthetic and a cocktail of painkillers don't lend themselves to movement in a patient.

Although it was July, it was Ireland, so it was lashing rain, windy and, after the dry heat of the hospital, it felt freezing.

Cian had parked in one of the ambulance spots at the main entrance, which is a hanging offence. He was met by an irate doorman. Now, I could understand the boiling fit of rage had we dumped our vehicle in the middle of two spaces and gone to the pub for the day. I know it's selfish and dangerous to obstruct the passage of the emergency services. Cian hadn't pulled in there hoping to aid and abet the death of an innocent patient. The stooping, green-tinged person in the wheelchair made it blatantly obvious we weren't there for a bit of diversion.

All I can say is that if I hadn't been in so much pain, I know I would have had one of those *Falling Down* moments. You know that movie where Michael Douglas's character has just had enough? He gets out of his car and marches into his local burger joint. When his burger doesn't look remotely like the one in the photo on the overhead board, he flips.

I found myself thinking like a character from a Quentin Tarantino movie. I narrowed my already slitty, drug-fuelled eyes. 'You need to calm down. I've had part of my innards removed only a few hours ago. I'm feeling sick, sore and more than a little bit pissed off. There are no ambulances here, there isn't a queue of five with people bleeding to death and sirens sounding like a bad version of a Scooter song. So do me a favour and either help us, or get lost.'

I know it wasn't polite. I know there was nothing ladylike about it, but I have never claimed to be a lady, and I can always blame the drugs if the same man ever meets me again and tackles me over my behaviour.

Cian had a whole other agenda to cope with. I couldn't stand up, so he needed to shift me from the wheelchair to the car. That might not sound like an enormous issue, until you take the logistics into account. At the time Cian was the proud owner of a sky-blue vintage sports car. It was unarguably a thing of aesthetic beauty, and was petted and admired everywhere it travelled.

But when you've got an immobile wife who's just been partially filleted, it's not the most suitable mode of transport. It was so close to the ground that it was difficult to sit into at the best of times. It required fairly strong thigh muscles and the ability to swing your head down and under, unless you wanted a whack on the noggin. Eventually Cian managed to fold my aching, slumped, sack-of-wet-sand body into the passenger seat.

Pain and trauma seemed to manifest itself in an angry sort of way that day. I wasn't even close to tears. Nor was I feeling sorry for myself and thinking, 'Why is this happening to me?' Instead I had an unquenchable urge to go on a dreadful rampage and inflict damage on inanimate objects. Not very Christian of me, but that was how I felt.

Every pothole, speed ramp and bump on the way home caused me to moan. I would have yelled loudly, and even used foul language, had I not been drugged to virtual silence. My outburst at the porter had used up all my reserve energy. Luckily we work as a team, Cian and I, so he did enough cursing for both of us.

By the time we made it to Bray, I felt like I'd spent forty minutes in a tumble dryer. Cian had put the heating on full in the car, not wanting me to be cold. I was so stoned, I couldn't tell him my organs were beginning to stew with the heat. The bone-shaker sports car, lovely to behold, was as cushioned as a slab of marble. Thankfully the children were in bed. I would have hated them to see me in such a bad state of disrepair.

Chapter 11

Ruby Slippers

We all have moments in life when we wish we could fly. Be it that day you're dying for the toilet and traffic won't move, or that moment when your flight has been cancelled due to a technical fault. All those reasons would have paled into insignificance in comparison to that car journey. I would have used up my once-in-a-lifetime chance to have grown wings that day ...

Before, during and after my surgery, the biggest incentive I had to press on and keep fighting was my children. My husband and family are my first priority. I know I am blessed to have their love and support. In turn, I feel I owe it to them to stay alive. They are the reason I never tire of fighting.

The family-in-the-garden arrangement has worked very well for us. Although Mum and Dad are a wonderful support, they don't infringe on our privacy. From the word go, when the children were babies, we always had our own babysitters. Apart from the fact that my parents have a better social life than most teenagers, we have never expected them to put their entire lives on hold for our children.

That is not to say that Sacha and Kim don't tell tales on Cian and me regularly. If we both say no, they'll inevitably sneak next door and try to extract what they want from Oma or Grandad. So we have a swift texting system in place, for example:

Do not agree to buy that new Wii game. We have said no.

Close-proximity living works for our family. Another wonderful advantage to living beside my parents is that we 'share' two dogs. 'Share' is a loose word, purely because my mum does all the work, i.e. walking and feeding the dogs, yet they come across to our garden and we get to play with them. We are what one might call à la carte dog owners!

The night Cian brought me home after the oophorectomy, my old childhood bed beckoned. I couldn't face the thought of the children standing beside our bed in the morning, looking at me worriedly as I tried to mask raw pain, so I figured the best solution was to go back to my mum and dad for a bit. Cian carried me up the stairs and Mum tucked me in as Dad made me a cup of herb tea. The familiarity of my old Laura Ashley print curtains, my white-painted iron bed and the small window of being a daughter again, instead of a mummy, was what I needed.

I will never tire of acknowledging that I am one of the fortunate ones. I have a husband, parents, family and numerous friends, who are always on tap and willing to help me. The public hospital system wouldn't have given a toss whether or not I was going home to a shoe box on the side of the motorway, with nothing but a dog on a piece of string to keep me company. I remember shuddering at the thought of not having professional care that night. What about the people who didn't live in their parents' garden? What about the people who didn't have anyone to curse at and lift them in and out of a car? It depressed and scared me in equal measure that many people must be sent away after surgery in a similar state to mine, but with no backup at the other end. We are meant to be living in a progressive modern society. Why does our public hospital system lack the ability to protect patients?

My ovaries were removed by keyhole surgery. When surgeons in general talk about keyhole surgery, there is a suggestion that it isn't going to hurt much. All the surgeons need is a tiny access area to ram and poke around. Whether you end up with a zip the length of your body or just a few stitches, it doesn't determine the post-operative pain, however. I had been lulled into a false sense of security. 'You won't have many stitches – it's keyhole surgery. You'll be right as rain in a jiffy.'

Lies. All of it. Do not be fooled: minimal gashes don't mean you're not going to wake up feeling like you've been violated with a pair of hedge clippers. I found the ovarian surgery more painful post-op than the double mastectomy. I often wonder if part of the reason was shock. With the mastectomy, I braced myself for dreadful pain. I imagined I would be shuffling around like a landmine victim. But the oophorectomy was a short space of time on the operating slab and a tiny scar. That couldn't possibly hurt. Oh yes, it bloody can. Since then I haven't had any preconceived ideas of exactly how I'm going to feel after surgery or treatment. It's very hard to change your mind when you haven't factored in the aftershock.

The children were a tonic as usual. Although Sacha and Kim were most definitely mini technical wizards, with an inbuilt ability to program gadgets, every now and then they still did childish things. Kim had this wonderful old-fashioned habit. Apart from the count- less emails and text messages I received from both children, Kim still made cards. Most nights, she used to put a little card or drawing between our pillows, with messages of love: 'Dear Mum and Dad. Thank you for being nice today. You are the bestest Mum and Dad in the world. You are both very good at being mums and dads. I love you. Sleep well. I hope you dream about me. Love Kim.' Or it might be a heart cut out and coloured in rainbow stripes, and then doctored hugely with 'magic pens' (yes, I did buy them from the ad on the telly – those ones that can transform colours with the stroke of the white 'magic' marker) and 'I love you' written on it.

To say that Kim went into overdrive when I was sick is putting it mildly. She barely had time to eat or go to school. The playroom would turn into a Hallmark-style production centre. Of course, I kept all these cards in a drawer and some will appear at a later date, like on her wedding day. Sacha only ever did art at a push, because in reality he preferred to shoot the heads off soldiers in a war game on PlayStation. Even at that stage, though he was only six by then, he'd moved away from the point in his young life where colouring held any appeal for him. So when both of them arrived into my old childhood bedroom with stern faces, each clutching a handmade card, the alarm bells rang.

'Are you not going to be our mum any more? Are you back being Oma and Grandad's little girl again?' Kim asked.

'Can we come to the sleepover tonight?' Sacha asked, with tears in his eyes. 'You've had two sleeps here and we miss you. I even made you a card.' He held it forward, offering it to me solemnly.

That was it. Enough of lying in bed. Enough of giving in to the pain. Time up. Besides, I had the two biggest hurdles behind me. Nothing in the world can jolt me into action like my children. Once I saw that they needed me at home, a missing limb, the fires of hell, mountains and oceans wouldn't have kept me away. That was it. I was through to the next round of the game. I had collected enough sympathy points, I had wallowed past 'Go' and I was on the home stretch – literally.

Chapter 12

Sympathy?

Pain, wallow, waddle – sympathy for self? So last week. Let's go to the baby shop. Why did I have to remove the parts that are difficult to explain to small children? It would have been so much simpler to get rid of a toe …

So I hobbled through the old stone archway, which looks like a porthole to Fairyland, between our house and my parents'. I vowed not to grimace or stoop too much. I decided I was better. Come hell or high water, I was back on Mummy duty.

I believed in being honest with my children in an age-appropriate manner. So when I had my breasts removed, I used the 'bad beads' analogy.

'I have some beads living in here.' I'd placed the palms of my hands over my breasts. 'Daddy and I and the doctors are worried that the beads are going to turn bad and make me sick. So the very kind and clever doctor is going to take them away,' I explained.

'Is it going to hurt you?' Sacha had asked.

'Oh, no, I'll be fast asleep.' I smiled.

'But what if you wake up? Will it hurt then?' Kim wondered.

'No. You know the pink medicine you get when you're not well or if you have a pain? Well, the clever doctor has a really good one of those and it makes any sore pain go away. It even makes you go to sleep and have gorgeous dreams. When I wake up, all the badness will be gone away,' I promised.

'But what if the bad beads roll on the floor and get into someone else?' Sacha's brain was working overtime.

'Ah, well, they've thought of all that. They have a special bag with a big knot in it. So the bad beads will go in the sealed bag in a big deep bin, where they'll never be able to hurt anyone ever again.' I nodded and looked into his eyes. 'I'm having this operation because I want to. Nobody told me I had to. But I want to make sure that I'm safe and that no badness can happen to me. Do you both understand?' I asked.

'Yes,' they chorused.

That was the first of many such conversations I had and still have with my children. But being honest and upfront from the start opened the door to them. I never wanted them to walk into a room where adults either stopped talking or mentioned something that frightened them. I hate being lied to. It upsets and infuriates me more than anything else in the world. I find lying pointless and hurtful. So I would never do it to my children.

When I had my ovaries removed, they were puzzled as to why my tummy was sore.

'Did you have bad beads in your tummy too?' Kim asked.

I know the quick, easy answer would have been yes, but then I would have had to revisit the issue and tell her the correct information at a later stage. I felt it would have been confusing and ever so slightly dishonest to lead her to believe that the mastectomy and oophorectomy were the same thing. After all, even toddlers are able to learn where their nose and eyes are. That delightful song 'Head, Shoulders, Knees and Toes' is a prime example of that very concept. I didn't want to be all 1950s about it and decide that because the body parts involved were 'wimmin's bits', I shouldn't name them. Let's face it, the children didn't give a hoot if I was talking about my eye or my arse.

'No, I had my ovaries removed,' I began.

'What are they? Can I see one?' Sacha asked.

'No. They used to live in my tummy here.' I pointed to my lower abdomen.

'What did they do?' Sacha asked, looking down at his own tummy. 'Where are mine hiding?' He was pulling up his T-shirt for me to show him the spot where his ovaries lived.

'They used to keep seeds in them that could come out and grow a baby,' I said. 'And guess what? Boys don't have ovaries, only girls.'

'Ah, so instead of ovaries I got a willy!' Sacha was clearly pleased.

'Exactly!' I exclaimed, thrilled he was understanding.

'Well, that doctor isn't cutting my willy off.' He folded his arms and looked as intimidating as a curly-headed blond six-year-old could manage.

Kim was peering through her long eyelashes with the concentrated expression she still assumes when a clanger is on its way out of her mouth. 'So when you were using the seed from the ovaries, did you put the seed in a pot like the cress in school?' she asked, hands on hips.

'It went into a special bag in my tummy called a womb.'

'And then it growed into a baby? So that's why mums get a fat tummy when they have a baby inside them.' Sacha looked like some jigsaw pieces were clicking into place for him.

'Exactly.' I was pleased.

'And how do they get out again once they've growed into a baby?' He wasn't letting this drop.

'Well, they either come out near the lady's bottom or out her sunroof.' I laughed.

'Where's the sunroof?' they chorused.

'That's the little space the doctor makes in some ladies' tummies if the baby can't come out near their bottom.' Needless to say, this evoked squealing and giggling until Sacha's face grew visibly troubled.

'What are you thinking now?' I coaxed.

'Well, if your seeds are all gone, then you can't grow any more babies to come out your bottom or your sunroof. So how are we going to have more brothers and sisters to play with?'

Before I could even begin to answer, Kim had it all sorted. 'Why don't you ask Dad for a loan of a seed and we can plant it in your tummy then?' she suggested helpfully.

'That won't work, Kimmy. Remember, Dad has a willy like me, so that means he has no seed things,' Sacha informed her.

'So does that mean we won't be allowed to have any more children in our house at all?' Kim was quick off the mark.

'Yes, it does. But I'm not sad about that because I asked the angels for two babies, and guess what?'

'They gave you us – we know!' Sacha rolled his eyes. One of the soothing stories I told them if they were sad or tired, as I stroked their hair away from their foreheads, involved the angels. Years previously, I said, I had asked my friends the angels for two little babies. A boy baby and a girl baby. The angels were so kind that they made my wish come true. That was why I had my two children. By age six, Sacha was a bit bored with the angel story, hence the eye-rolling.

The conversation ended abruptly as the cat began to chase a feather around the garden. Their focus left me and my lack of baby seeds was passé.

As children have a wonderful ability to remember every conversation dating back to their second week of life, I knew that might not be the end of the subject.

Sure enough, a week later Sacha arrived into the kitchen with Kim behind him.

'Mum, we've been chatting.' He had his hands on his hips. Kim studied his stance and did the same. 'We've decided that the best thing to do is go to the baby shop in Vietnam.'

They know several children who have been adopted from Vietnam, but I had never referred to a shop.

'Oh, honey, you can't go to Vietnam and get babies from a shop. It's much more complicated than that. In fact, it takes years and years to get a baby.'

I was all ready with my politically correct version of adoption and how we should never say 'shop' in the same sentence as 'adoption'.

'But my friend is from Vietnam. She told me that her parents went there and they had lots of love and lots of money, so they put the two together and bought her.'

Sweat beaded my brow. His little friend had obviously decided this was how she'd made her way to Ireland, and from the look on Sacha's face, he was undeniably impressed with the whole concept.

'Was I bought at a baby shop?' Kim stared at me, willing me to say yes.

'No, lovey. I grew you in my tummy.' I smiled.

'Well, can we tell people that you bought me?' She bit her lip and looked expectant.

'Not really – and, besides, you look quite like me, so nobody would really believe you.' Luckily, the combination of an older brother when I was growing up and my familiarity with small children's honesty ensured I wasn't too sensitive!

'But I want to be from Vietnam,' Kim whined, pouting.

'Quiet, Kimmy, we're doing a deal, remember?' Sacha glowered at her, silencing her abruptly. 'Well, we've decided that it would be a good plan to go to Vietnam tomorrow. We'll help with the payment. Look.' Sacha emptied his piggy bank onto the kitchen table.

'I'll go online and book the flights,' Kim said. 'We know how to do it – we saw the ad on TV.' She nodded.

'They're doing flights for next to nothing at the moment.' She recited the ad she'd seen: '"The next new city is only a heartbeat away."'

'And I've agreed that we'll even take a girl, if we can't buy a boy,' Sacha sighed.

I had to pull every type of compliment out of the bag for both Sacha and Kim to reassure them that they were enough for Cian and me. And, more importantly, that we had no intention of buying babies or adding to our family.

'But how will we manage with only two children in our family?' Kim looked most perplexed.

'Well, we've managed quite well up until now, so I wouldn't worry about it, love.' I grinned.

In the end, I resorted to the age-old quick fix. Bribery – with the promise of a marmalade kitten. We already had Tom the cat and over the years he survived several kittens from tabby to marmalade. All perished while he continued to soldier on. Tom has chronic asthma and needs an injection once a month. Nobody thought he'd survive for long, but now, twelve years later, he's still here!

While the decision to end my fertility didn't cause me any lasting difficulty, and I have never had any regrets with regard to my actions, I am fully aware this is an enormous issue for young women without children. My theory that everything happens for a reason comes into play. We hadn't planned on having Sacha at the precise time he graced us with his presence, but once I was faced with the decision to have my ovaries removed, the reason he had been sent to us in 2000 became glaringly obvious. Equally my palpable yearning for another baby almost immediately after Sacha's arrival made sense. Something or someone was guiding me and making sure I had my family sorted before BRCA1 came crashing through the swinging double doors of my life.

Chapter 13

My Houdini Moment

Phew! Can't get much closer than this. I know how it must feel to miss the bus that carried the suicide bomber ...

In September 2006 Mr Geraghty, my mastectomy surgeon, called us into the hospital for a chat. The analysis of my breast tissue had revealed that there had been some activity in the left breast. The cancer party had just started.

To say that I hadn't been warned about this party was an understatement. If the cancer had had a brain, it couldn't have picked a better place to hide. It was forming right in the centre of my breast. Bang in the middle of the densest part of the tissue.

I had acted just in time. The pathology suggested that the cells could have been forming for more than five years – since Kim's birth in 2001. I wasn't large-breasted, at size 34B, but all the same, due to my age (thirty-three at the time), it would have been very difficult to find the potential tumour in my young, taut breast tissue.

I felt like the person who'd fallen asleep and missed the aeroplane that crashed and killed every person on board. It was like an out-of-body experience. A million thoughts went through my mind at once – relief, fear (fleetingly), gratitude and guilt. It all ended in slight hysteria.

It was such a narrow escape that I nearly thought I should do something mad, like run up Grafton Street naked, banging a large drum.

Now we all had justification for my actions. I knew from those results that I would never have a moment in the future when I thought, 'Why did I put myself through that surgery?'

The words that had been uttered to me echoed in my mind: 'You're not actually sick, Emma. Take your time. Look at all the women in this corridor alone. They've been diagnosed with cancer.' My God, was I glad I hadn't listened to anyone but myself. I say this to people until I'm blue in the face: we all know our own bodies. Never let anyone tell you otherwise. Trust your own instinct and don't deviate from that.

I was advised that no further treatment was required. I could skip away into the middle distance. Sadly, I was to discover that the middle distance was a lot further away than I had ever anticipated. Hindsight is a wonderful thing and, had I known what lay ahead, I would have demanded a scan at that time. But I naïvely believed I had side-stepped my biggest nightmare – cancer.

As Cian drove us home from the appointment that evening, I clearly remember calling my parents and his parents, followed by close friends. We all breathed a collective sigh of relief and, in a slightly dumbfounded way, agreed that I had escaped the worst by the skin of my teeth.

Chapter 14

Surgery Number Three

My boob job. Hope I don't end up looking like a total tit!

In October 2006 I went back to Tallaght Hospital to have implants inserted. Known as the 'exchange surgery', it was a straightforward procedure (especially if you're a surgeon!). It involved the removal of the expander bags full of saline and the installation of the silicone implants. As I described earlier, the expanders had been inflated with saline to create a pocket for the implant to live in. If that doesn't happen, the skin and muscle act like a claw, squeezing the implant and producing a puckered result.

By all accounts, this was going to be an easy-peasy surgery. In fact, I was so cavalier towards surgery by now that I could have had it done in the hospital shop on top of the ice cream freezer without pain relief. I was an accepted inmate on the surgery front and even knew some of the theatre staff by name. If they had operated a points system, I would have been in line for a free sandwich toaster, or even a set of bath towels.

As predicted, the exchange surgery wasn't awful. I was in very little pain afterwards. The area around my mastectomy scars had hardly any sensation because all the tissue, nerves and other connecting goo had been removed. I could probably do a circus act in which clowns hit my boobs with lump hammers, while I stand in my pink sparkly leotard wearing an unflinching smile. If things get really bad financially in the future, I'll keep it in mind.

I had to stay in hospital for a couple of days, as I had drains in again. But I was unfazed. The first time I'd gone to hospital, until I got to know the other inmates and the general running of the ward, I was afraid to leave my bed and found the dynamics of the place terrifying. This time I was doing laps around the corridors, and trotting in and out of the shop almost as soon as I came to from the anaesthetic. All I was missing was a set of wrist and ankle weights, a pink towelling headband and a plastic bottle of water.

Besides, I was jumping the final hurdle. I had taken control of BRCA1. I had reduced my chances of developing cancer from 85 per cent to 5 per cent, as the research and statistics had shown. I was only short of holding my dressing gown aloft behind my head (if my arms hadn't been wrenched down after the surgery) and doing laps of honour, while waving and high-fiving passers-by. Cue blue-birds tweeting, a meadow of brightly coloured flowers and a happy ever after.

Chapter 15

A New Dawn, a New Day, a New Year!

Tiny alarm bells are ringing in my head. My eating habits haven't changed, but my thighs are expanding at a rate of knots. Is this the dreaded menopause? Aaagh! I'm only thirty-three!

Christmas 2006 was like Mardi Gras at our house. We were all on a high. It had been a long, tough year. Although we'd all seen enough hospital corridors to last quite a long time, we knew it had been worthwhile.

The surgery, instead of being a negative concept, had offered me the highest prize – life. By going ahead with the operations, I had chosen to live.

Santa was very good to us. A new machine called a Wii was unleashed upon the world. Every man, woman and child wanted one. Like many others, Sacha had asked Santa for a Wii. As they were about as available as hobby-horse poo, I'd sort of assumed that Santa would have to write a letter saying that, due to overwhelming demand, there would be a bit of a wait for the Wii to be delivered. But, purely by chance, I happened to be in the toyshop when a first-come-first-served unexpected delivery landed.

Sacha was ecstatic, and the fever took over our entire house. In the beginning we joined in with the children simply because it was the right thing to do. Very quickly it became apparent that this new console was going to cause divorces and broken friendships across the globe. Competition was fierce. The newspapers were reporting an influx of injured, inebriated adults in A & E departments the length and breadth of the country: determined and bloody-minded parents were wrestling the controls from their children and falling over coffee tables in the hope of beating a child or Yuletide visitor at Wii golf. Cian and his cousin Garrett stayed up until five in the morning on New Year's Day, playing 'just one more game' of Wii bowling.

As well as Santa coming that year, I think we all felt like we'd been visited by angels too. As the New Year bells rang, we clinked our glasses and heaved a sigh of relief. Although I was certainly glad to bid farewell to 2006, I also felt an enormous sense of satisfaction. I had jumped all the hurdles I had set for myself. I had exercised my determination and I had achieved everything I had set out to do that year. That is a wonderful feeling, believe me.

But then destiny stepped in. My life took a very different direction, one that I would never have imagined in my wildest dreams.

By the end of January 2007, a niggle was gnawing away at my mind. I wasn't feeling quite right. I had been quashing the thought for a few weeks, but as time moved on, and I knew I should be over the surgery trauma, my euphoria was fading. For ages I was afraid even to tell Cian. The fact of the matter was that I felt like shit. Straight up. When I eventually fessed up during the third week of January, Cian was pragmatic and not too alarmed.

'Give yourself some time. You've just had a full-on year of surgery. You're not the Bionic Woman. You just need to have that thing you've never heard of – what's it called again? Oh, yes, patience.'

'Ha-ha, so funny.' I grudgingly had to admit that I felt a bit cheated by my lethargy. I had expected to feel inspired and energetic and able to take on the world. I should've been Maria from *The Sound of Music*, filled with song and arm-waving in my frilly apron.

Instead I was exhausted and gaining weight at an alarming rate.

The glaringly obvious problem and the one that made the most sense was menopause. I'd had my ovaries removed and the doctors had explained that I would be thrown into a 'medically induced menopause'. Unlike the natural menopause, it occurs literally overnight.

At the age of thirty-three, I knew very little about the menopause, bar the fact that women got hot flushes and some of them went a bit doolally. 'Isn't this the time where rich women get arrested for stealing lipstick from chain stores and end up in court as a sobbing mess, apologising to a judge who looks uncomfortable and lets them off with a week's community service and a wagging finger?' I mused.

'And that's why there are so many older people raking and replanting at roundabouts all over the country,' my friend Jade agreed. She had called in for a cup of tea and some sympathy.

'Do you think I'd get away with robbing a Chanel handbag and a matching wallet?' I suddenly felt brighter.

'No, I can't see that working too well. Besides, you'd probably have to bring all sorts of papers to court to show you actually are hitting menopause. You're hardly the stereotypical Menopausal Mindy to look at, now, are you?'

'Oh, yeah, I forgot that. So are you saying that I'll have to wait another forty years before I can get away with shoplifting?' I asked Jade. 'Why are you looking so suicidal?'

'Your hormones, or lack thereof, are in direct contrast to the rampant and murderous ones I'm attempting to deal with here.' Jade looked down at her swollen belly as she sat drinking mint tea and dabbing her eyes as her head rushed with pregnancy-driven madness.

'You'll be back to normal as soon as that baby is born. I could go on being a lunatic for years. At least you have a timescale to work with, not to mention the reward of a baby at the end of it. And you're not planning on getting arrested so you're in a win–win situation,' I assured her. I pushed the plate of brownies towards her.

'The only saving grace is that starving yourself isn't going to make you look any better, so you might as well spend all your waking hours eating all the things you usually deny yourself.'

'There's nothing more creepy than skinny pregnant women,' she shuddered.

'I agree – it's right up there with emaciated babies. Infants are supposed to have rolls of soft squidge, with little elastic-band type wrists. When you're a baby or the baby-growing vessel, it's OK to be huge.' I nodded and patted her hand, while simultaneously shoving a brownie at her.

'Thanks, Emma. God, I'd say you're glad you're not a waddling ten-ton-Tessie, like me,' she sighed.

For a split second, I felt a tiny tug inside my chest. Was this regret coming to test my resolve? Did I feel sorry I would never be pregnant again? Was I suddenly going to yearn for a baby to hold? Was I going to change my mind and decide I needed more children?

I waited and held my breath. I closed my eyes to allow myself to concentrate. It could have been the faint sound of a heartstring. Ping! That was it. Then I looked at my usually svelte friend, an inflated version of herself, and I was cured. 'You've it all ahead of you, my girl.' I grinned. 'All the nappies, sleepless nights, world falling out your arse after the birth. Ah, the joys.'

'Shut up – you sound like an auld one!'

'I feel like an auld codger, to be honest. Menopause is a disaster. So enjoy your rampant hormones while you still have them. Mine have all drained away. God, I feel woeful.'

I gave up attempting to have menopause conversations with my own friends. They just couldn't imagine how it felt. Which was fair enough. I began quizzing all Mum's friends instead.

I had hoped menopause was a bit like the baby thing, that it was this kind of informal club, and once you tapped into it, people would start to tell the truth. But when I scratched the surface, no information poured forth. Maybe it was my mother's generation of women or maybe they didn't know a whole lot about it, but I was getting nowhere – fast.

I knew there was the HRT approach, but I'd done so much medical stuff and doctors and hospitals, I wanted something gentler. There was the stick-waver business, which involved eating bits of forest floor and taking wheelbarrow loads of unpronounceable drops from tiny glass bottles, but that seemed a little too eye-of-newt. I figured my local health food store might be a good place to begin.

'I need some menopause-curing stuff, please,' I stated hesitantly.

'Pardon?' the person with knitted everything and many rings in her nose answered.

'Menopause-removal magic dust, please.' I smiled.

Mrs Scrubbed-with-a-Brillo-pad and not a screed of make-up looked out from under her bushy monobrow at me. 'For you?'

'Yes.' I wasn't in the mood for telling her about the last year and how I was now feeling worse than before.

'Right.' She looked at me suspiciously.

'It's been brought on prematurely due to medical intervention. I'm hardly looking to take menopause stuff for a kick,' I reasoned.

'Of course.' She didn't smile and kept looking back over her shoulder rather crossly.

I probably should've walked out. Instead I had to bite my tongue. I had an awful urge to yell, 'If I was in line for doing something a bit mad, don't you think I would've gone to a head shop and asked for the herb version of heroin? Stop looking at me in that tone of voice.'

I left with a thin brown paper bag, which was splitting under the weight of the boxes and drops. I knew that no trees or worms had suffered to make that bag, but it was as much use as an ashtray on a motorbike. Furthermore, the whole lot had cost me a small fortune. If it had all tumbled onto the footpath and smashed, I would've been forced to kneel down and lick it all up.

Alternative, my eye! Uncut cocaine would have been cheaper. Just because it's made from all natural stuff and is put into tiny bottles, they seem to think it's all right to charge the same price as a weekend in Paris.

And a couple of weeks later I wished I'd opted for the city break instead. I felt worse. Any energy I might have had was dwindling rapidly. I spent half my day measuring drops and downing tablets the colour of compressed moss. There didn't seem to be any magical cure for this nasty sluggish feeling. All advice pointed towards HRT.

'It was the answer to my prayers. Once I found the right one, I was flying,' one of Mum's friends confided.

Fantastic! I'd be as nimble as a mountain goat, with the constitution of an ox. Simple! I felt much brighter than I had for weeks and thought all my problems would be solved by a prescription. Easy, right?

No. Not quite. I discovered that there are a million and one forms of this HRT stuff. Liquid, patches, pills, injections, creams, natural, organic, alternative, and the list goes on. I returned to the gynaecological surgeon in Tallaght. I had seen him a couple of times since my operation for post-surgical check-ups, and he'd indicated that I should wait a few months before taking HRT, to allow my hormones to deregulate. My lack of energy, hot flushes and generally down-trodden feelings were telling me I was well and truly deregulated.

The doctor I ended up seeing was not the most approachable person on the planet. He wasn't one for big chats, explanations or even eye contact. I dubbed him 'Piehole' because he was disinterested, lacking in empathy and one of those gits who believed he was God. Giving him a derogatory name made him less intimidating and made me feel like less of an idiot in his company. As he chewed the top of his pen and sighed while looking at his watch, I explained how I was feeling.

Piehole scribbled a prescription, then sneered, 'Try it for a couple of months. You might need to try a few before you find the one that works best. Shut the door on the way out.'

Ciao, Piehole, smell you later. Hope you step in dog poo on your way home tonight, I thought to myself.

Almost immediately, I developed a rash. At first it was only notice-able in certain lights. I returned to see Piehole. He kept me waiting for more than two hours and was sarcastic, virtually yawning in my face as I spoke. 'I'm covered in a rash, I feel dreadful and I can't think of any reason for the symptoms other than the HRT. Can I try another one?' I asked.

'Yup. Although I doubt the tablets are causing the rash you're speaking about,' he barked.

'Well, the rash is pretty obvious – it's on my face and arms, as you can clearly see,' I began.

'Right. Try these and come back if they don't work. Give it a while, though.'

The rash got worse. It crept from my scalp down the tops of my arms, across my torso and down my legs.

I returned to Piehole. He wasn't available, so I saw the doctor on duty. He barely looked at me and I was prescribed yet another brand of HRT.

By this stage, I had developed an added annoyance. I had begun to bleed. Feeling really stupid and scared, I rang the hospital again.

'Is it normal to bleed during menopause? I assumed I wasn't supposed to have periods any more,' I hesitated.

I was put on hold, passed from one person to another, and eventually told to come in the following day.

I was greeted by yet another strange face.

'We've never met, but come this way.' A white coat flashed and I assumed I was to follow this new doctor, who had a thick foreign accent and an apparent lack of spare time to converse with me.

I stumbled up the corridor after him, then found myself in a room with a chair like a dentist's.

'Please remove the bottom half of your clothing and we'll perform an internal scan,' a young nurse explained.

I did as I was told and perched on the seat nervously. The examination wasn't painful, but it was as relaxing as having pins poked in my eyes.

'There doesn't seem to be a problem. You'll need to take a tablet to coagulate your blood and a different HRT.' The doctor did some scribbling and made a quick exit.

It took a few days for the bleeding to stop. To this day I have no idea how or why I bled at that time. Nobody explained, and I was too miserable and exhausted to ask.

The rash was still raging on. By now my face, upper torso and thighs were red raw. I was getting nowhere with the medics so I tried to find another way to cure myself – one that didn't involve annoying any more doctors or being made to feel like an annoyance.

I quite honestly had no idea what was wrong with me. I did wonder whether it was my body rejecting the breast implants. I'd heard stories of women having boob jobs and discovering they were allergic to the silicone. But the hospital reassured me that that sort of reaction was extremely rare now, because implants and plastic surgery had become so sophisticated.

Still, I knew the way I was feeling wasn't right. Our lives should have returned to normal. The children were settled back in school after the Christmas holidays, Cian was working and I should have been well on the road to getting everything back on track. I should have been at the point where I was able to talk about my surgery and my brush with BRCA1 in the past tense.

Not sure of what to do next, I turned to the Internet. After diagnosing myself with everything from meningitis to scabies, I did the obvious. I went back to the alternative medicine expert. Of course I did.

'Your body is rejecting all the fabricated chemicals in those hormones. You need to see a Chinese doctor. Someone who specialises in natural things,' said the knitted person.

By now I felt utterly despondent. I felt like I was banging my head against the wall – and my rash was getting even worse.

So along I went, and met a gorgeous person who stuck needles between my fingers, toes, skull bones and every other place I really didn't want her to. As I lay there, thinking, 'Please don't put them in my shin – that would be really vile and sore,' hey presto, there were four in it. I can't say it hurt, but the idea of it was just dreadful.

'Just lie there and relax,' she said soothingly. Believe me, it's not that easy when you look like a porcupine made from Meccano.

Then came the bags of stuff from places like the Congo basin and the northern tip of Saturn. 'You'll need to boil them up, strain the juice and drink it three times a day.' It could have been leaves from a rare bubblegum bush and a dash of teddy-bear saliva. All I knew was that chemicals were the devil's spawn. My body was reacting to them and I needed to 'clear' my system. I dutifully went to an eco shop and spent the mortgage money on shampoo, shower gel and washing powder made from natural ingredients.

The rash got even worse. Added to the hideous itch, which was so bad I had to tape socks to my hands at night to stop me scratching, my arms and legs were so sore. The bathroom smelt like the jacks on Bray seafront, and the children had dandruff from the 'special' shampoo.

Every morning I felt like I'd danced till dawn while drinking straight tequila along with the contents of the slops bucket at my local bar. I know it's dreadfully vain of me, but when the rash crept all over my face and I put on three-quarters of a stone in one week, I knew I had to do something. Other than when I was pregnant with Sacha and Kim, my weight has always been pretty much the same. I wasn't eating lard for breakfast – there was no normal reason why I would suddenly gain so much weight. That was it. I had to get to the bottom of exactly what was going on with my body.

Chapter 16

Not Just an Itchy Face

I am not feeling well. Things must begin to improve quick smart or the next stop needs to be the vet or the nuthouse. Either will do.

It was May 2007. I had spent the guts of six months being driven demented, going in and out of hospital, boiling potions and doing everything I could think of to make myself feel better. None of it had helped. I was struggling to carry out everyday duties. Raising my arms to wash my hair was difficult and painful beyond belief. My hands had almost seized up. Brushing Kim's hair and putting it in pigtails was nearly impossible. Tying shoelaces or zipping up a jacket were tasks I used to take for granted. Now I struggled to do them at all.

I reached a turning point one morning when we were getting ready for school. Kim had a ballet display that morning. She wanted a pink ribbon woven into a plait in her hair. My hands were so stiff and sore, I couldn't make my fingers bend around the hairbrush. I had to phone my mum and ask her to come and help me. We both knew there was something significant going on, but probably because I was in a rush, not to mention within earshot of both children, neither of us adults said too much. I attended Kim's little ballet display and made my way to the supermarket.

Lifting the shopping bags from the trolley to the car made me cry out in pain. I now know that someone was smiling down on me and guiding me at that time.

'I can't do this any more. I'm not happy being a metal hedgehog with pins being stuck in me constantly and I've had enough of gagging on stewed vegetation tea,' I whined to my friend Corina that very afternoon.

'Why don't you try and get something done with the rash at least? That way you'll start to feel better. My brother-in-law is a skin specialist in Blackrock Clinic. Let me call him and see what he thinks,' she offered kindly.

Her brother-in-law didn't like the sound of my rash or my piling on weight without the aid of pies. He offered to see me the following day.

Cian decided to drive me, just in case there was anything wrong. I'd say at this stage he was fit to strangle me, what with all the surgery, the constant trotting in and out of hospital, chopping and changing HRT, not to mention the blasted rash. What could possibly be wrong now?

Corina's phone call changed my life. Dr Cal Condon is a skin wizard in Blackrock Clinic in Dublin. He had never seen me before, so he had no proof that I didn't usually look like a boiled chipmunk after a fight with a Black & Decker sanding machine. As he greeted me, I got that look. It was fleeting, and in Dr Condon's defence, very discreet. But I clocked it.

'What?' I demanded, squinting at him suspiciously.

'You're very ill.' He looked me straight in the eye.

'Thank you.' I exhaled and smiled. Now it was his turn to look shocked.

'You don't understand,' I went on. 'I've spent the last six months trotting in and out of hospital, telling anyone who'll listen that there's something wrong. Until this second, nobody believed me.'

Deep down, I had known for months that there was something wrong. I was glad I hadn't allowed myself to be fobbed off. I was glad I had gone to another doctor and another hospital. That second opinion was to save my life.

Dr Condon kicked into action. He took a skin biopsy on the spot. He ordered a nurse to take what felt like an entire pint in blood samples and advised me to go home and rest. 'I'll be in touch quickly. You won't be left wondering where I am,' he promised.

Unlike the others I'd seen, this man meant action. He was friendly and warm and polite, but I knew he meant business.

I probably should have gone home fretting from Dr Condon's office. On the contrary, I was relieved. I just knew he was going to find out what was going on and have a good go at helping me. The most terrifying and isolating part of my illness came to an end once Dr Condon took over. Until that moment, I felt like I was (a) a nuisance, (b) a hypochondriac, (c) going insane. I hadn't ever striven to be any of the above. But the fact that I had asked questions over and over again and had met with a brick wall each time had led me to feel I must be wrong. If I was genuinely sick, surely it would have been spotted. Self-doubt had crept in, and even though I was finding it difficult to conduct my daily life, I had come to think that I ought to feel that way. Pain and discomfort and itching had become the norm.

To have another individual stand in front of me and not only believe me when I said I wasn't well, but also vow to help felt like a miracle. I was walking on air – well, in reality I felt like I was shuffling painfully through treacle, but you know what I mean.

Within a couple of days I found it hard to walk and raise my arms upwards. The only way I can describe it was that I felt like the Tin Man in *The Wizard of Oz* when Dorothy first meets him. It was like my joints had become rusty and immobile. I was virtually bedridden. The pain in my limbs was excruciating. My face, neck and shoulders had inflated so much I looked like an American football player – except I wasn't wearing any added padding. Two small rubber peas had appeared in my neck, just above my collarbone.

The blood samples were taken on a Thursday. Dr Condon phoned me the following Monday morning.

'I'm going to admit you. There's something serious going on here and we need to start running further tests immediately,' he advised.

At last I was being taken seriously and listened to.

I will never forget walking into the main hospital that day. I was met by Carol on the front desk. She filled in forms and brought me to my room. The muscles in my arms and legs burned with raging pain as I eased into a pair of pyjamas and sank into the hospital bed.

Right at that moment, if a team of vets had come into the room and informed me that I needed to be put down, I don't think I would have argued. Without a shadow of doubt, that was the lowest point of my entire existence. I sincerely hope I never feel such turmoil and anguish again.

Chapter 17

Feeling a Bit Pea-ed Off

Captain Birdseye has nothing on me. Only the best peas make it to the pathology lab. I also think I may have an idea for a new book – 101 uses for a staple gun.

My slippers may not have been of the ruby variety, but somehow (you know the way some people do insane stuff at night and have no recollection of their actions next morning), I must have clicked my heels three times, because the Blackrock Clinic was as close to home as a hospital could be. A whole new world of medical marvels opened up to me. Blackrock Clinic is a hospital but it's run like a business. That might sound wrong to you but, believe me, it's right on so many levels.

No doctor, nurse or specialist walks into your room without being briefed by the manager on duty. The files are held at the main desk of each section. The manager explains everything to every doctor who walks into your room. Gone was the Groundhog Day behaviour I had experienced over the previous six months. In fact, the tables turned so far that the doctors who came to see me actually offered their services. They volunteered information on how they felt they could try to help me. They also seemed to have a policy of not making patients feel like they were interfering with their day. They knew phrases like 'How are you today?' and 'How are you feeling?' and 'Does this hurt?'

The pain in my limbs was so bad I was on heavy-duty pain medication, muscle relaxants and steroids. I was so swollen and red that my family and friends had gone beyond the stage of pretending I looked fine. Instead, they'd come and visit, stand dumbstruck at the foot of my bed and let the bag of sweets, magazines or other thoughtful gift slip to the floor.

'Holy shit, what's happened to you?' they'd exclaim. Thank God for honesty. If they'd come in and told me I looked great, I would have mustered up what strength I had left to throw them out. For future reference, it's just the same as telling a pregnant woman who is a week overdue that she looks 'very neat'. Don't do it. Either say nothing or go for: 'Bet you can't wait for it to be over.'

I still remember comforting a sobbing friend, years ago, as she poured her heart out over her impossible-to-shift post-baby weight: 'It was bad enough that I had to stand on the talking weighing scales at the top of the room. But when Mags patted my hand and told me not to mind it, that I looked really skinny, I wanted to throttle her. I've never been so fat in my entire life. I've put on even more weight since I had the baby,' she sniffled.

I felt my friend needed honesty at that moment – and who better than I? 'That Mags one shouldn't even be allowed at WeightWatchers. She's only there to give everyone else a complex. Listen, you do look like you've eaten all the pies. You've never looked like this before, but you can lose it. You can get back to the way you were. I did.'

Now, you're probably thinking what a bitch I was. I should have done the 'kind' thing and said she looked gorgeous. But I knew she was miserable. She didn't want to look the way she did. She'd never looked that way before. It's like clothes-shop assistants who tell you everything you try on is 'gorgeous', when you know you look like you got dressed in the dark in someone else's clothes.

White lies when you know you don't look the way you should create a feeling of inner fury. Don't fuel it. You don't have to say, 'Jesus, you look like a corpse/Weeble/freak,' but perhaps lay off, 'You've never looked better in your life.' While I was looking utterly scary and bloated and red, I found comfort in people I loved and trusted telling me they thought I looked like something from Elm Street.

'At least I don't usually look quite this shit, so maybe I'll resemble something normal again soon,' I ventured.

I could have opened a serious gift shop with the proceeds of all the presents loved ones brought me. It never ceases to amaze me how thoughtful, generous and kind people can be. I was busy putting on hand cream and sniffing the matching shower gel, propped up on clean pillows in brand new pyjamas, with fifteen magazines and a nest of boxes of chocolates, when Dr Condon knocked on my door.

'I know what's wrong with you.' He sat beside my bed. 'We suspected lupus at first, but the bloods have shown it to be dermatomyositis.'

'Dermato-who?' I couldn't even say it, never mind attempt to figure out what it might be. It's a ridiculous name, and sadly it doesn't have funky initials – I can't hang out in Starbucks and nonchalantly drop the fact that I've got DMY.

Dermatomyositis is a rare disease that turns the immune system on itself. Its symptoms are:

1. An itchy, burning, raw rash on the arms, legs and torso. Hence the rubbed-by-a-dry-loofah-for-far-too-long look.
2. Seizing up of the muscles, with pain similar to arthritis. Hence the movements like the Tin Man's and being as nimble as an arthritic geriatric.
3. Change in voice pitch. I had been feeling like a teenage boy. My voice had been fluctuating from normal to deepest bass.
4. Difficulty in swallowing. A really odd thing had begun to occur. Every time I drank anything, hot or cold, it came out of my nose.
5. Rough skin on the hands. My nail folds had yellowish hard and painful skin around them. I also had the violet rash on my knuckles.

'OK, so what do we do about it?' I leaned forward. 'Just as long as you can stop the pain and get me walking properly, I'll do anything.' The pain, straight up, was worse than childbirth without an epidural. It was constant too, whereas the labour pain stops the second the baby arrives.

'Dermatomyositis,' Dr Condon spoke slowly and clearly, 'can occur on its own or in conjunction with cancer.'

My hand instinctively flew to my neck. Fingering the two rubber peas, I held his gaze.

'We have to biopsy them to see what's going on in there.' He looked worried.

Blackrock Clinic is unique. I can say that with plenty of evidence to back it up. I have done a pretty impressive tour of various hospitals at this stage of my life, and I have yet to find a place that runs as smoothly. When they say they're going to do something, consider it done. Immediately. Coupled with the fact that Dr Cal Condon is a total perfectionist and a man who gets things done, I was in the right place.

Mr Magee was brought on line. He removed the rubber peas and they were sent off for testing.

As you can appreciate, myriad emotions were running through my entire being. The constant flow of well-wishers and visitors was welcome during the day. When they had gone and I was left alone to my thoughts, I needed time to take stock of what was happening.

I ran a bath one evening, figuring it might be relaxing and might even help with my aching limbs. I can probably count on one hand the number of times I've sat in a bath over the last twenty years – no, I don't smell of foot rot, I'm just a shower person. The idea of wallowing in my own skin flakes never appealed to me. There's also that body-morphing thing that happens, where your legs look like they're more deformed than normal, and your wobbly bits are all magnified. I lashed in a load of bubbles, hoping to avoid the 'Oh Christ, do my thighs really look this bad?' syndrome. As I lowered myself into the steaming water, the tears began to flow. I closed my eyes and braced myself. If I was diagnosed with cancer, I had to accept it and move on. I willed myself to have the courage to fight this disease.

'Mim and Helen, if you're listening, help me, please,' I said aloud to the ceiling, begging my friend and my aunt to look after me.

How did I feel, deep down inside? OK, actually. This was the thing I had removed body parts to avoid. This was the situation I had dreaded ending up in, more than any other. But I'd had a strong feeling that I was going to find out I had cancer anyway.

A million scenarios flew through my mind. Sacha's first communion the following year. I'm not remotely religious, but I didn't want him to have to sit in the church with no mum. Christmas. Their birthday parties. Who else would bake them a mud and worms cake? Who else would spend hours surfing the Internet for trinkets to put in going-home bags? Who would make sure they didn't have matted hair and clashing clothes on to go out in public? Who would sew the name tags onto their school uniforms? Flying further forward to the future: who would help Kim pick her wedding dress? Who would be the mother-in-law from hell to Sacha's wife?

Tears had begun to fall from the second I sat in the water. As I pictured my children progressing through the important stages of their lives and the milestones that I hoped they would make, I forced the tears away. Who would do all those things? I fucking would. That's who.

I wrapped myself in a towel and made a conscious decision to rise above it. I promised myself I would do everything in my power to stay alive. I had tried to avoid getting cancer. I had done my best. But if destiny had decided I was to battle it anyway, well, the fight would begin.

The determination that surged through me at that time was a physical as well as mental sensation. It was a different feeling from my determination to have the mastectomy. That had been my own doing and my own choice. If I was to be diagnosed with cancer, it obviously wouldn't be my choice. I wasn't in a position to call the shots. But one thing was for certain: I might not be able to decide if I should get cancer, but I could sure as hell decide how I was going to deal with it.

The following morning Cian brought the children in to visit me.

'Mum!' They rushed like excited puppies and leaped onto my bed, oblivious to my swollen face, red rash or obvious discomfort. Hugging them to me I knew that they were the final kick in the pants I needed. Looking at their animated faces as they told me in unison every move they'd made that morning, what they'd eaten for breakfast and how Dad had promised them a chocolate muffin if they behaved at the hospital, I knew I was lucky.

Nothing in the world, no disease, surgery or tragedy, could destroy the pure joy my children brought to me.

'Mum, there are metal things in your neck! Who did that to you? That's very dangerous!' Kim shrieked.

'Mum, let me see.' Sacha was up on the hospital bed, with his face stuck in my neck.

'They're staples. I had some rubber peas living in there and nice Mr Magee took them away. My neck was a bit sad because he took its peas, so he gave it some cool staples to play with for a few days.'

'Are they sore?' They looked worried for a second.

'No, actually they're not.' I wasn't lying. 'But before you get any ideas, these are special medical staples. You're not to go home and staple Kim's foot to the carpet, you hear?'

They giggled and we had a wonderful conversation about stapling people's eyelids open, or getting mean people and stapling them to the curtains. The children left thinking staples were a hoot. It was immaterial that I looked like Herman Munster's sister or that I'd just had a bit of my neck removed.

I did text Cian on the quiet and insist he search the house for any staplers and put them in the wheelie bin quick smart. Whatever about the children, I feared for the safety of Tom, our faithful old cat.

Chapter 18

Derma Who?

What? Ah, come on, lads, can't we just change the name to something easy, like Bob or Maud?

It was the beginning of June 2007. I knew I had a big disease with a very long name. But until I met my next specialist, I didn't really know what I was supposed to do about it. Enter Dr Frances Stafford, rheumatologist. We met for the first time at eleven o'clock at night. She knocked on my door and apologised for the late consultation. A petite, ladylike woman, she deftly examined me and made notes.

Dr Stafford has one of those personalities that lets you know she's in control. She's as gently spoken as a fairy, with tiny hands and dexterous movements, and exudes knowledge.

I immediately felt safe and trusted her. Yet again, I was being linked up with a professional who believed me and promised to help me feel better.

'This is a fairly rare disease, but I have seen it before,' Dr Stafford explained. 'I'm going to start you on a hefty dose of prednisolone. This is a steroid that I hope will begin to arrest it.'

She moved my arms and legs, bending and pushing, figuring out how much movement and strength I had. The answer was none of either. 'You'll need physiotherapy to get those limbs moving again – I'll contact the department. They'll be in to you tomorrow.' She smiled.

When Dr Stafford left my room, I had to sit in the quiet for a little while, so I could take all the new information on board.

I phoned Cian. Even that was difficult now: my arm was so swollen and the muscles were so tight, I couldn't actually keep my elbow bent or hold the phone up to my ear. Luckily I had the attachment with the earpiece and microphone to plug into my mobile. That was the only way I could even use the phone.

'Hi – are you OK?' He sounded groggy.

'Sorry. I forgot it's so late. I just met a rheumatologist called Dr Stafford,' I began.

'What? At midnight? Where? In a pub?' Cian was very confused.

'No, she came in to see me and explained all about dermato-myositis and prednisolone,' I buzzed.

'Who, what, where?'

'Yeah, I know, we need an episode of *Sesame Street* brought to us by the words "autoimmune disease" with the special word being "prednisolone". It would help if I had a disease with a name that's easier to pronounce, not to mention treat.'

'So what does this prednisolone do?' Cian was wide awake now.

'It's a steroid and it basically goes in and stops this autoimmune thing in its tracks. I've to take a really heavy dosage at first, and once things improve, I can gradually wean myself off it.'

It sounded simple and I hoped it would work. Never having taken steroids before, I had no idea of the side effects they brought with them. For the first while, the disease was so advanced that the effects weren't too harsh. I think the steroids were so busy hammering the dermatomyositis on the head, they didn't have a chance to cause me too much grief. But over a period of time, as they built up in my system, I began to suffer with insomnia. To counteract that, I started taking sleeping pills.

I had gone from a person who boiled up vegetation instead of taking medication to a walking drugs cabinet. Oddly enough, I took comfort from the treatment. Don't imagine for one second I was glad to be a legal druggy – not at all – but there was a sense of safety: I knew I was being monitored and the medication was being prescribed to do a good job. If the hospital had told me opium sandwiches would improve my health, I would've eaten them.

Chapter 19

Knock, Knock

Who's there? You won't believe this but …

Exactly a week after Mr Magee had removed the rubber peas, Dr Condon came to visit again. I was still in my room in Blackrock Clinic. The high dosage of steroids was making my already puffy exterior look like rising yeast dough.

Dr Condon sat down with his takeaway cup of coffee. Some people have a security blanket or a perpetual cigarette in one hand. Dr Condon has a cup of coffee. I knew before he spoke what was coming. 'I wish things were different. There's no easy way to say this, so I'm going to be direct. You have cancer, Emma.'

Slowly and calmly, I gazed out the window. My bedroom looked onto a secondary-school playground. A group of girls, wearing itchy restricting uniforms were sitting on the tarmac surface. There they were, totally unaware of me watching them. They all stood up, brushing dust off their clothes, and reluctantly made their way inside the building to begin their Leaving Certificate exams.

'God, I hated exams,' I stated, still watching the girls' retreating backs.

'Pardon?' Dr Condon followed my gaze.

'Don't have me carted off by the men in white coats, but I'd rather be in here, in spite of what you've just told me, than in their shoes, walking towards an exam hall.'

'Are you OK?' Dr Condon leaned forwards in his chair. 'Did you hear what I just said to you?'

'I knew all along,' I admitted.

'I know you did.'

There was damn all either of us could say. That was that. I had known. The minute I'd been told there was a connection between dermatomyositis and cancer, it had made sense in my head. The jigsaw had clicked into place.

It was like the day I had gone to Nuala Cody for my genetic test results. I had known I would be gene-positive. I'm not Mystic Meg. Neither do I think I have untapped powers to heal wounded animals and cure lepers. But I believe we all have an inbuilt knowledge of ourselves. Most of the time, thankfully, we just don't need to use it.

'I have to pass you on to an oncologist now. It's not my field. I'd like you to speak to Dr David Fennelly. He's a friend and colleague. I know you'll like him and he's very good at what he does. Unless there is someone you particularly want to attend,' he said.

'I don't hang out with medical specialists, unlike you, so I'll take your word for it. If you like him, I'm sure I will too.' I grinned. 'Thank you for taking the shitty end of the stick.'

'What do you mean?' He looked puzzled.

'You could have sent Dr Fennelly straight in here to speak to me, but you didn't. You knew you were being handed the shitty end of the stick and you took it. Thanks for coming in and breaking the news. I couldn't do your job.'

The news wasn't great: I had been told I had cancer. That's pretty bad in the greater scheme of things but I was struck by the choice Dr Condon had made. He had opted to come and deliver the blow. Take a second to imagine you're a doctor. However awful it feels to be told you have cancer, can you imagine being the one who has to let the patient know? Sod that, I could never do the job these incredible specialists do. All the brains in the world and all the hours of medical school cannot make a person compassionate.

I had seen doctors who didn't believe me, others who looked down their noses at me, making me feel I had the brainpower of a slug, for daring to ask questions. Dr Condon had turned all of that around for me. It was like that moment in *The Wizard of Oz* when the screen turns from black and white to glorious colour and the Munchkins begin to sing.

It's always easier to hear difficult news from someone you know. That day I was glad to have Dr Condon carrying the shitty stick! Thank you, Cal.

OK, the news could have been better, but the colour button had been adjusted.

So, how did I feel now? Was I pissed off? Hell, yes. Was I surprised or shocked? Hell, no. As I said, I had known. For the week that I'd sat in that hospital bed awaiting the test results, I'd known it would be cancer.

Was I upset? Of course I was – I wouldn't have been human if I hadn't had a rush of fear and sadness. I allowed those emotions to wash over me. I didn't feel hysterical. There was no urge to lie on the floor yowling like an injured animal. I didn't burst into tears, thump the wall or shake from head to toe. Instead I was accepting of my diagnosis. It was almost a serene feeling. The one thing I had feared so terribly had come home to roost. I can only compare it to the day I started my Leaving Certificate exams. From the moment we start school, we are being primed for this one set of exams. All the tests leading up to it are geared towards this big final blowout. The pressure mounts and the years, months, weeks and eventually days pass until the big day finally dawns. Once the exams have been completed, whether or not you have done well remains to be seen. But I had finally faced my demon. I had completed my exams. I felt a huge sense of personal accomplishment. Equally, when I was pregnant for the first time, I fretted for nine months about whether or not I would be capable of giving birth. When I did it twice, my God, it made me feel a thousand feet tall.

Cancer had been the gremlin on my shoulder for a long time – since my aunts had been ill and especially since I'd known about BRCA1. Now, finally, in June 2007 it was D-day.

Once the doctors and nurses left my room, I took a few moments to gather my thoughts. I remember clearly being OK with the whole thing. What I wasn't happy about was telling my nearest and dearest. They were waiting for my results. Each of them would be going about their day as I sat and pondered. It was my job to phone them in turn and shatter them. Believe me, that isn't a nice job. Knowing the news had to come out, I braced myself.

I phoned Cian. 'Can you talk?' I asked, my voice wobbling.

'I'm just buying work uniforms for the lads. Can I call you back?'

It was probably the familiar sound of his voice, but I couldn't wait five seconds longer. I had to tell him. 'I have cancer.' I promptly burst out crying.

'OK. We'll do this. You'll fight it. Hold tight. I'll be there in a few minutes.' He hung up. He told me afterwards that he'd turned and run out of the shop, calling over his shoulder that he'd be back later, there was an emergency.

As soon as I hung up, Mum's number came up on my phone. 'Hi, Mum!' I heard my two children shouting in unison. She was bringing them to school, and they were ringing from the car to say good morning. That was one of the hardest moments of my life.

First, I wanted to tell my mum. When you're sick, you tell your mum. But my heart was being torn in two as I heard my children's voices, happily shouting into the speakerphone. I should have won an Oscar for my performance. I took a deep breath and grasped the sheets of my hospital bed with both hands. I had the earpiece for my phone installed and I gulped as I tried to control my voice.

'Hi, guys, how are you both this morning? I hope you ate your breakfast.' I closed my eyes and begged for the strength to hold on to my control. They shouted at the same time about the day ahead.

'I'm going on my school tour to the zoo,' Kim chirped.

'Of course you are, honey. Silly Mum forgot. What did you bring for your packed lunch?' I rubbed my forehead. Luckily Kim was more than thrilled to tell me exactly what she had.

'How are you, Sach?' I asked my son.

'Good. When are you coming home?' He sounded less cheerful.

'Soon, darling, I promise.' My voice was beginning to crack. I wasn't sure how much longer I could continue the false cheer.

'Sacha is just a little sad because Kim is going on her tour today, but I've promised him we'll make cake when he comes home later on,' Mum interjected.

'OK, you guys, have a fun day and call me later on to tell me all about the zoo, Kim. Sacha, you take a photo of the cake you bake and send it to my phone, OK?' I was breathing heavily. 'Talk to you all later.'

'Bye, Mum!' they yelled, pleased that they had the makings of a good day in prospect. I hadn't been able to tell my mum my news. There was no way I could blurt it out while she was driving, and I needed to work out how to tell the children.

I made a few more calls, to my dad, brother, cousins, Cian's parents and close family members. As I waited for Cian to arrive, I sat in the silence of my hospital room. I couldn't turn on the television. I couldn't take any noise or distraction. My mind was whirring. I was trying to swallow the fact that I had cancer. Yet at the same time I knew so little about what was going to happen. It was an odd feeling of limbo. I felt like I was floating in the air, drifting between moments of disbelief and acceptance.

I sat and stared at the wall. I grabbed my diary. My hands were so stiff and sore from the dermatomyositis, it was hard for me to write. Here is my diary entry on that day, word for word:

It's Wednesday, 6 June 2007. I have cancer. The thing that I fought to avoid. The one thing I dreaded most of all. In spite of all I did, I've got it anyway. I will fight this. Now that it's visited me, I don't feel so bad. It's not as dreadful as I feared. I don't feel like it will beat me. With God as my witness, I will fight this bastard every step of the way. Bring it on.

As I wrote, I felt more empowered by the second. The fight was on. I was utterly determined I was not going to lose. I'd come too far to go backwards. It was obviously my destiny to have cancer. The odds on me getting breast cancer were so low, after all I had done. But I'd got it anyway. Cancer is a seriously complex disease and just because I'd taken all of the safeguarding measures available to me, it was never going to guarantee I would always be free of the disease. I had just hoped that would be the case.

Many of us have heard of the stages of cancer. These are based on the size of the tumour, and the purpose of the staging system is to help the doctors to sort the different factors and some of the 'personality features' of the cancer into categories. I had metastatic cancer, which meant that the cancer had spread beyond the breast and nearby lymph nodes, even though this was the first diagnosis of breast cancer. The reason for this is that the primary or first part of the breast cancer was not found when it was only inside the breast. Metastatic cancer is considered stage IV. This is what I've been diagnosed with each time. At the risk of sounding like a frustrated medical student, I'll explain the stages of cancer in more detail and in my own words in a section at the end of the book – for those of you who like that sort of information!

So the way I saw it was this: it was meant to be.

If this was what I was put on this earth to do, I was ready.

By the time Cian made it to the hospital, followed closely by my parents, I felt less terrified and calmer. As they crowded around my bed and we chatted about how much of a pisser it was that I had got cancer, the thing that has kept me going over the years began to pour forth: laughter.

'Do you think I would make the front page if I rang one of the tabloids? I can see the headline right now – "Bray woman gets breast cancer even though she has no breasts".'

'That's not funny.' My mum looked stricken.

'It is a bit funny, really.' I grinned. 'I think I'm kind of talented, even if I say so myself.'

There were plenty of silences that day. We were all stuck for words. Even though we are always the 'noisy table' in any restaurant when we go out together, even though we have the ability to make each other cry laughing at the most serious of times – that day, laughter was almost absent.

Cian looked exhausted. My parents seemed to have aged since the day before. My cousins Robyn and Steffy left work and came over to see me. They were upbeat and encouraging. My older brother Timmy came in – a feat in itself. Over the years he had spent his fair share of time in hospital with Crohn's disease, so he doesn't 'do' hospitals unless it's totally necessary. In spite of the crowd and the shoehorning of bodies into my room, we all had little to say.

'Well, the worst-case scenario has happened. At least we've got that out of the way,' I observed. That in itself was a sort of release.

'All we can do now is gather as much information as possible and deal with it,' Cian said.

'We all know you'll fight this, and we'll do what we can to help,' Mum said.

I had every intention of fighting – there was no doubt about that – but I felt something else: guilty. I felt so bad that I was putting all these people I loved through such heartache and worry. I didn't feel sorry for myself. I felt sorry for them. They'd all dropped what they were doing and appeared in my room so I could see their concern.

When I'd phoned each of them early that morning, I didn't ask them to come in to see me. I'd delivered my blow and we'd finished our conversation. They all appeared one by one, gravitating towards me and engulfing me in their love.

I may have been told I had cancer. It mightn't have been ideal on lots of levels, but I most certainly wasn't alone. For that, I will be eternally grateful.

Chapter 20

How to Get to Oncology Street

'Hi children, today's programme is brought to you by the words "rheumatology", "dermatomyositis", "prednisolone", "tumour" and "cancer". Come and join us — it's going to be so much fun to learn together.'

As I mentioned before, one of the worst parts about being diagnosed was the dilemma of how to tell everyone. From extended family to friends, there were suddenly so many people I had to inform. Many people choose not to tell anyone if they're ill, but that's not my style. I couldn't keep this monumental news to myself. I would have shrivelled up and died on the spot if I'd had to carry the burden of cancer on my own. I needed to share my problem. I needed to tell people. I just wasn't sure how.

I wanted the children to know before anyone else. I didn't want them to be told by someone else in a way that would worry or upset them. I asked for them to be brought into the hospital so I could tell them. I figured if it came from me and I looked and sounded positive, it would soften the blow. After all, I was their mum: they trusted me. I was nervous as I walked from my room to meet them.

It was 9 June 2007. They met me in the hospital's coffee shop, and we settled at a table with juice and chocolate muffins.

'The reason I have a funny rash and have to do sleepovers in the hospital is because I have two things wrong with me,' I began.

Their legs swung as they munched the muffins and stared at me comfortably.

108

'What is it?' Sacha asked, as he picked the chocolate chips out of his muffin (to save for afterwards 'cos they're the best bits).

'One is called cancer, and a man doctor called David is going to fix that. I haven't met him yet, but I hear he's a great guy. The other is called dermatomyositis, and a lady doctor called Frances is going to fix that one.' I smiled.

'That's fair, isn't it, if both a boy and a girl get to fix you?' Kim nodded.

'The cancer has given me some little lumps called tumours. But now they're all gone away – that's why I had the operation. It's much better to have the tumour removed,' I tried to explain.

'What's the tumour's name?' Kim wanted to know.

'Cancer,' I explained.

'We know that, but he must have his own name – the tumour, that is.' Sacha was obviously on the same wavelength as Kim.

'What would you like to call him?' I played along.

'Henry,' Sacha decided.

'Yup, that's OK,' Kim agreed.

So tumours were referred to as 'Henrys' from then on, *chez nous*.

'So, back to the medicine and the doctor.' I tried to keep them focused for just another little minute. 'Do you know the funniest thing about the cancer one?' I raised my eyebrows and gestured for them to lean in close for the secret answer.

'What?' They both grinned.

'The medicine is going to make all my hair fall out!' Luckily they saw the funny side of this and giggled loudly. (The really unfunny part about losing your hair to chemotherapy is that all your body hair – yes, all your body hair – falls out, except the hair on your legs. How bloody unfair is that? So I was going to be as bald as a baby and still need to have my legs waxed!)

'Noooo way! That's cool.' Sacha shook his head and raised his shoulders, giggling some more.

'Can you come home soon, Mummy?' Kim looked at me intently.

'Very soon, lovey, when the doctors know how much medicine I need to make the bold diseases stop annoying me.'

'When you come home, can we all go for ice cream?' Sacha wanted to know.

'You bet we can. I'm looking forward to it already.' I held my arms out and they both leaped off their chairs, scattering bits of chocolate muffin for miles around.

An elderly couple sitting behind us had overheard our conversation and were sniffling uncontrollably.

'Why don't you two go outside to the little decking part with your juice? I'll put the muffin wrappers in the bin and follow you,' I suggested.

They were gone like puppies before I could even finish the sentence.

'I don't mean to interrupt, but I know you overheard my conversation with my children just now. I'm sorry if I upset you. I thought it was better to say the word "cancer" and just be straight with them.' I bit my lip.

'Don't you worry, dear. It was a sad but lovely thing to overhear.' The elderly lady patted my hand. 'You're so right. In our day, nobody was encouraged to talk about these things. Too many awful and sad things were pushed under the carpet. You do right letting those little angels know what's happening. You did it so beautifully too. May God watch over and protect you.'

As soon as the children knew about my cancer, I felt happier. Little people are so incredibly accepting and adaptable. They hadn't learned the art of lying yet either.

The hospital informed me that I would be introduced to David Fennelly, my oncologist, later that day. He would fill me in on the plan of action. But seeing as I have zero patience, I did what most computer-literate people do: I googled dermatomyositis and cancer. Yes, I frightened the living daylights out of myself and, yes, I diagnosed myself with at least fifteen further illnesses.

We've all done it. Found a link, clicked, clicked on the next bit, and ended up with a random list of symptoms we apply to ourselves. I ended up feeling paranoid and panicked. I terrified myself so badly that I shut the laptop and decided to listen to my own human medical team. After all, they'd been to medical school and had studied oncology and rheumatology, so logic would indicate that they should have known what they were talking about.

My room was like the upstairs of a pub all afternoon. Family, friends, doctors and nurses flooded my space. All that day, the nurses popped their heads through my door constantly. 'Hi, love, just checking how you're doing. How's the head space?'

'I'm good so far, thank you. I don't need to be on suicide watch yet. In fact, you can write in indelible pen that I won't be trying to top myself. I'm planning on doing the exact opposite.'

That evening, my door opened slowly. A bunch of flowers was held aloft just inside the frame. Then Ruth and Cathy jumped in – my two aunts who'd survived cancer all those years ago. Both are still very young, I would like to stress. The auntie label conjures up a slightly stereotypical image. For the record, these two are the utmost in style. Not a moustache or hairy mole in sight.

'We're here to show you we're not dead.' Ruth grinned.

'We brought you flowers, to show we're giving them to you now, not on your grave.' Cathy beamed.

They were exactly what I needed. No doctor or specialist could have made me understand survival like the two living, breathing and very young aunties. They pulled up a chair and gave me a good talking-to.

'OK, I get it.' I laughed. 'So, dying isn't an option. I've to endure the chemotherapy and put on the boxing gloves.'

Being part of an entire family of girl-power people, from Oma down, has helped make me the person I am. Defeatist talk has no place in a cancer diagnosis. The medical findings on the results with patients who choose the positivity route are astounding. Case studies have shown that a cheerful outlook, coupled with the correct medical intervention, can catapult even the most grim prognosis to a better level – a 30 per cent higher survival rate has been reported among patients with a positive outlook.

On Thursday, 7 June, I had met Dr David Fennelly for the first time. He's a consultant oncologist or, in plain English, a cancer slayer. Although he doesn't wear full armour or carry a shield and sword, I reckon his middle name is secretly Excalibur.

I didn't know what an oncologist was supposed to look like. In my mind's eye, I guess I must have thought he'd be something like the crazy-eyed fella with the mad wispy white hair in *Back to the*

Future. But David Fennelly was none of the above. Not a protruding eyeball in sight.

I instantly felt at ease with him, and he welcomed my barrage of silly questions. (Some of which I'd downloaded from mentalers-r-us. com.) 'Because I have dermatomyositis, does that mean the cancer is in my organs too?' One particular website I had encountered had illustrated that the autoimmune disease could occur concurrently with lung cancer.

'We honestly don't know yet, Emma. We're going to do some scans so we can figure it all out,' he explained.

'There's no rule set in stone that I won't survive this, is there?'

'Definitely not. There's always hope.'

The fact that Dr Fennelly wasn't looking like the Grim Reaper and grunting in answer to any question I asked filled me with confidence and hope. Surely if the whole situation was utterly bleak, this man wouldn't be smiling.

'The first step is a PET scan. This is a very sensitive machine that shows us layer by layer what is going on in your body. We'll know what's happening with every inch of you once the images are through.'

I asked an alarming number of questions about the scan. The full name is 'positron emission tomography' – but PET sounds much more fluffy and less scary. It would take a couple of days for the scan to be set up and for the funding to be cleared by my health-insurance provider.

I didn't have the energy to call each and every person I knew, so I sent a text. That sounds so cold and shocking as I write this, but I felt it was the quickest and easiest way. I wanted my diagnosis to be out in the open. I didn't want whispering and curtain twitching. But most of all, I didn't want the cancer to silence me. If that happened, I personally felt it was one up on me.

Dear Friends. I'm sorry 2 tell you all this via text & apologies 4 the group message. Sadly I have been diagnosed with cancer. Scans in 3 days. Will keep u all posted. I've come 2 far 2 bow down now. I will beat this bastard. Emma x

The three days I had to wait seemed like a year. Every time I sneezed, coughed or twitched, I wondered if it was due to a brain or kidney tumour, a liver invasion or an entire body attack. Now that I knew every layer of my body was going to be looked at, I wondered how much cancer was festering inside me. Would I be told I had a month to live? Would I turn out to be one of those unfortunate people who would make it into the Guinness Book of Records for harbouring the most impressive number of tumours in one single body at one time? Was this the reason why I had put on weight so swiftly? Was it because the tumours weighed so much?

I had dreams about snarling hairy yokes with crooked teeth exuding smoky brown steam and talking to me in a creepy way.

'Who are you?'

'We are cancer monsters. We are eating you from the inside out.' They sneered horribly.

I'd wake up sweating, needing a few seconds to realise it was a nightmare and that my mind was playing tricks on me. I fixed the problem by taking strong sleeping pills. I can't say they made me sleep well – they simply obliterated me and made sure that I conked out and went to a place where my imagination wasn't allowed to function. If I woke during the night, I had no recollection of it. The last thing I remembered was turning off the television. Then the lady was there with my breakfast tray, opening the curtains. That suited me perfectly. It wasn't a time of my life that needed full glaring reality shining through twenty-four hours at a time. The few hours of drug-induced blankness were a blessed relief.

For the first time ever, I could understand, even in a flickeringly brief way, why people become drug addicts. I had a whole new understanding of people who were dependent on substances. Maybe in the beginning the alcohol or drugs or whatever poison they favoured numbed their pain too. I'm definitely very fortunate that too much wine gives me such a vicious hangover: I have learned not to drink myself to oblivion. If I hadn't, I reckon I'd be a serious alcoholic today. As for the drugs – well, I've taken enough by mouth and through my veins to scratch that itch too!

Chapter 21

PET Hate

I love cats. So that's a sign I'm going to love this PET scan, isn't it?

The morning of the PET scan dawned. I was brought fasting to the Nuclear Medicine Department, which I thought was a marvellous name. I was expecting men in white space suits and ten-tentacled Cyclopses to do what had to be done. Instead I was met by a human in the form of a nurse. She didn't beep or use V signs with her green-podded hands. She didn't even have a silver necklace, let alone an entire boiler suit made out of tinfoil à la *Deep Space Nine*.

'OK, Emma, the first thing we need to do is inject some radio-tracer into your arm.'

'Ooh, that sounds a bit exciting. Will I look like I'm illuminated by one of those ultraviolet lights in a nightclub? Will I have really brown skin and bright white teeth?' I ventured.

'Sadly, no, the impact is inside your body. All this means is that I'll inject some contrast into your vein, which will adhere to any cancer that might be present. In turn, this will light up for our scanner.'

So, the bottom line was that it was a sort of magic cancer-highlighting dye. No disco look, no ultra-bright smile. Ah, well.

'You need to lie as still as you can in this room and we'll come and get you for your scan in about forty minutes. I can happily stay with you if you're feeling anxious.'

'Why do I have to lie still?' I wondered.

'The machine is so sensitive that it picks up on any recent activity. It's so responsive that we've had a reading where a patient had a whole block of colour across her shoulder and upper torso.'

'Jeez, was she riddled with cancer?' I was horrified.

'No, she'd been carrying her baby. The child had fallen asleep with her head on her shoulder, and the entire area had lit up afterwards. So we need to you lie still and try to relax. Will I stay?' the nurse asked kindly.

'No, I'll be fine, thank you.' I was handed a remote control and a pile of magazines. I didn't want either. I closed my eyes and spoke to the two people I always called on.

I am baptised Catholic, but I don't believe in any form of organised religion. I don't attend any form of religious service. But I do believe in spirits. I do think we all go to a form of paradise when we leave this world. And I know that the people we love are still with us.

I take comfort in chatting to my loved ones who've gone before me. Perhaps I will be locked up for this at some stage, but so far nobody has caught me or had me assessed for doing it, so I'm safe enough. That day, I asked Mim and Helen to help me, to surround me and watch over me. The downtime flew, and before I knew it, I was being called.

'OK, Emma, follow me. Let's get your scan going.' The radiologist led the way.

The PET scanner turned out to be one of those in-the-tunnel contraptions, a huge white machine, housed in a spacious shiny room. The walls, floors and ceiling looked like an ad for kitchen cleaner. I reckon even the most anal housewife with white cotton gloves wouldn't find a speck of dust in that place. There was a table-style bed on a runner, a bit like a bobsleigh. Not a patch of fur or a paw in sight, sadly. This PET neither purred nor licked me.

'You lie on the bed and it moves by itself towards the open-ended tunnel. If you feel claustrophobic or panicky, just press the buzzer. The machine will stop and the examination will be cut short,' the radiologist explained. 'Try and remain as still as you can.'

The room was quite cold. The bed was quite hard. The whole thing was stark and white. But it wasn't scary. There were no big needles or mad-looking garden tools that looked like they could decapitate me.

'Would you like silence, or will I put on some music for you?' a voice came over a loudspeaker.

I resisted the urge to giggle and ask the mysterious voice if he was the Wizard of Oz. 'Music would be good,' I answered.

'Perfect, here goes. Just try and relax, Emma.' Unfortunately the album of choice that day was Dido. Even at the best of times after two bottles of wine, I find her on the whiny side, but, having listened to her during a PET scan, I have a whole new hatred for her music.

I survived the torture of Dido and her suicidal lyrics and the go in the scanner. Then it was back to waiting once again. The results would need to be analysed and scrutinised before my medical team could come up with a plan of action.

Meanwhile, I was still being given steroids to deal with the dermatomyositis. I was in so much pain, I still hadn't been home. I had been in hospital for three weeks, and even though it sounds odd, I knew it was the best place for me. It took me an hour to have a shower. I could still barely dress myself. Everyday tasks like putting on the washing machine or sweeping the kitchen floor would have been out of the question, let alone taking care of the children. I missed my babies so badly, but I was also cripplingly aware that I was of no use to them until I began to improve.

Most days Cian or my parents brought Sacha and Kim in to see me. Needless to say, they loved my hospital bed, which was electronic and made vaguely *Star Wars*-type noises. There were always sweets and boxes of chocolates dotted around the room, courtesy of generous visitors. My temporary home was south-facing so it would become as hot as a sauna.

'I'll bring you in a fan,' Cian promised.

'You could have a pet reptile in here, Mum. They love being in hot tanks like this. I know because I met them at the zoo,' Kim pointed out proudly.

'Fantastic idea, but I don't know if they allow chameleons in hospitals, lovey.'

Three days after my scan, Dr Fennelly came into my room with a big orange cardboard folder. 'I have your PET scan results here, Emma.'

'Did I pass?'

'With flying colours.' Dr Fennelly smiled.

'Despite Dido.' I grimaced.

Dr Fennelly looked momentarily puzzled. 'It's not important,' I assured him.

'Emma, you have cancer in your neck, where the rubber peas had resided, in your shoulder cavity and also your left auxiliary, otherwise known as your armpit.'

'Sorry for being so narrow-minded, David. But work with me here: how is that good news?'

'Because it hasn't spread to any organs. It's what we call a nodal invasion, so we can treat it very successfully with chemotherapy.'

Straight off, I thought of old-style Space Invaders. The ones that come in a block of about fifty little feckers dancing across the screen, and you're the little cannon firing bullets at them.

'So, what are the odds of you and the chemotherapy winning with this nodal invasion?' I asked.

'The chemotherapy and you are going to beat it. The nodal invasion is toast. Your chances of recovery are very high. Once the cancer is contained, we have very high hopes for you.'

Smiling is always a good thing, but especially so when you're talking to an oncologist. Not just because it's pleasanter, but you know it's for a good reason. Facial expressions are key when you're dealing with doctors.

The day I met Dr Condon: no smiling. The day Dr Condon had to break the cancer news: no smiling. PET scan results: smiling.

'Let the fight begin,' I vowed, as I shook hands with David Fennelly. The bet was on. I just knew we were on the winning side together.

I was so fortunate: my doctors were wonderful right from the off. They spoke to me like they really believed I had a brain. There was no smirking or head patting while they smugly assured me I was on a need-to-know basis. They were a fount of information, open to questions and fully confident they would help me beat the cancer and the dermatomyositis.

I trusted my doctors. I believed them when they said I could beat the illness. I didn't allow myself to go down the slippery slope of self-pity. I would stand up and walk around the hospital if my head started to melt. If I had the dark thoughts of my children having no mother, my husband having no wife, or my parents having no daughter, I would pound the floors. Well, I would haul myself out of bed, struggle to tie the belt of my dressing gown with my swollen sore fingers and do an aged-person shuffle around the corridors.

Like a lonely crazy person, I would smile like a loony and chat to strangers. I often bought packets of jellies from the dispenser machine in the lobby at four in the morning. I hate jellies. But there was nothing else. Besides, anything was better than going to the dark recesses of my mind.

If the shuffling around didn't work, I would give myself a stern talking-to. I sincerely hope they don't have a camera in the lift in Blackrock Clinic. If they do, I'm on it, muttering and wagging my finger at myself. I would make myself stand and face the mirror and I would say out loud in a firm teacher's voice: 'Stop it. No wallowing. You will be fine. This is not the end of the road for you.'

If my lip began to wobble, or my eyes even attempted to get teary, I would become a tough-love psychologist: 'Millions of people are diagnosed with cancer all around the world all the time. So why not you? OK, fair enough, I've gone to fairly extensive lengths to avoid it, but as the old cliché goes, there's nothing certain in this life but uncertainty. Good. Glad we've had this chat.' I'd wave at myself in the tinted mirror.

In time, I taught myself to think positive thoughts. I simply put a mind block on the negative. I was certain of one thing from that time forward: I couldn't control whether or not I got cancer, but I could sure as hell control how I dealt with it. It was not written in stone that I had to lie down and die. There were no rules when it came to coping with cancer, so I vowed I was going to do my own thing. I was going to beat the cancer with the help of my doctors. But more than that: I was going to do it with a bloody big smile on my face.

The cancer was NOT going to win.

Chapter 22

What Is Chemotherapy, Exactly?

Captain's log: chemotherapy day one, June 2007

Before I had cancer, I had no idea what chemotherapy really was. OK, I knew it was cancer medicine, and that people got sick, bald and had a deathly complexion.

The day I began chemotherapy, I was filled with mixed emotions. I was nervous, scared – and a little excited. The nosy part of me was looking forward to finding out what chemotherapy actually was. I didn't know what sort of a device they used. Would I stand up, sit down, lie on a bed, be strapped to a rollercoaster-type thing?

All I knew about cancer was terrifying sickness and sometimes death. Yes, Ruth and Cathy and many others had survived, but I hadn't lived in their homes or their heads during treatment. I honestly didn't know what to expect.

So when they wheeled in a small boxy unit, with a smooth keypad attached to a metal pole, I was a bit disappointed. 'Is that it? No curly wires or large noisy machine like a giant's hoover to suck my brains out?'

'Sorry, this is it. I'll bring the chemotherapy in in a minute and then I'll explain it to you.' The nurse smiled.

Oh, right, I thought. Now I need to brace myself. The chemotherapy will be in a huge freezer box, like the ones for organ transplanting, with dry ice wafting out of it. It will glow in a throbbing green-to-blue sci-fi-movie way. They'll lift it out while they're dressed in puffy white suits and padded oven-glove yokes on their hands for protection. This must be where the drama unfolds.

I eyeballed the innocuous machine. There were four little hooks at the top of the pole, which was about six feet high. The keypadded box was halfway down, with numbers, like an alarm system. I tentatively poked the keypad. It swung open to reveal rivets to attach a wire. At the back there was a black power lead.

Shortly afterwards, the nurse returned with two bags. One was about the size and shape of one of those Capri Sun drink pouches and the second about three times that size.

'OK, Emma, the small one goes first – it's the anti-sickness stuff. And the other is the first of your chemotherapy medications. Today you'll have three different bags of chemotherapy.' She placed the chemotherapy in a bright purple plastic bag and hooked it onto a little hanger at the top of the pole.

'Is that it? Just bags of liquid?' I must have looked crestfallen. 'No power tools or flashing lights? Not even a drum roll?'

'Sorry, pet, that's your lot.'

So, chemotherapy was a liquid – fair enough, a very potent one, but it was just a bag of juice.

Before they started the drip, Julie (who is a direct descendant of the angels, with her gentle manner and wonderful way of explaining even the most complicated things) introduced herself. She went through all the types of drugs I would be given, explained the possible side effects and gave me enough leaflets to wallpaper a semi-detached house.

I would receive most of my chemotherapy in the day unit, which was just down the hall, but due to my dermatomyositis and my general brokenness, I was having it in my own room to start with. I was to have a treatment every three weeks for six months.

'Is there anything else you'd like to know before we get you started?' I now know, after years of attending Blackrock Clinic, just how incredibly busy all the oncology team are – all the time. But that day, and any time I'm there, they have a wonderful knack of making me feel like I'm their only patient.

I learned that each time a patient has cancer, he or she must have a different mix of poisons. As this was my first time, I was getting the standard dose commonly used for breast cancer. 'So that means I would have to get different medicines if it ever came back?' I asked.

'Yes. The body can become accustomed to anything, and in a similar fashion, cancer can too. So we would need to use a different medicine to combat it.'

I was weighed carefully and had my exact height measured.

'Each dose is calculated according to your weight. It's worked out every single time you come for a blast. It's a major balancing act – too much would obviously run the risk of lasting adverse reaction; too little and the cancer won't be killed.'

This was one of those moments when I realised why we have to learn maths in school. I always hated maths and was one of those kids who thought, 'Why the hell do I need to know how much liquid a container that is "X" high and "Y" wide can hold?' Well, this was it. I was the container and they needed to kill the bad bits inside it.

'Will I be crawling around on the floor bathed in sweat and caked in my own vomit?' I asked.

'God, no!' Julie looked shocked. 'Emma, the anti-nausea medication is much more sophisticated, these days. If you ever vomit or feel really seasick, you must tell us immediately. There are so many forms of anti-sickness drugs that there is no need to suffer in that way.'

That made me feel much more at ease.

'One of the things the chemotherapy can do is burn the skin around the area where the needle goes in, so if you feel sore or see it becoming swollen or red, call us and we'll move the needle.'

I must confess to staring at the needle obsessively for the first few goes, wondering if it was doing anything awful. Believe me, when it does, you don't need to stare at it non-stop to know. I noticed another thing: all the medics I came across always called it 'chemotherapy', not 'chemo', as I'd heard it referred to.

'One of your medicines is called Adriamycin. It's bright red, so you'll pee red for a day or so. Don't be alarmed. It also causes alopecia. In other words, it makes your hair fall out.'

Ever since I was a child, I'd always had long blond hair. I'd never had a compulsion to shave my head as a teenager. I liked my hair.

Now I was faced with losing it, in the name of killing cancer. Under normal circumstances, I would claw you to death if you tried to shave my head, even for the most deserving charitable cause. I'm not that easy-going. But this was different. It was either long flowing locks or dead in a pine box. No contest.

'We have something called a scalp cooler. Riza is our resident expert on this and she'll tell you how it works. Would you like to talk to her?' Julie asked.

'Why not?' I shrugged.

Riza explained that chemotherapy affects all cells in the body, not just the cancer. It's like an internal full body wash. Places like the stomach, the lining of the mouth and hair follicles are especially sensitive, as those cells multiply rapidly. Cancer works the same way. It multiplies at a rate of knots.

'We offer a "cold cap", which is like a tightly fitted frozen swimming hat. It reduces the blood flow to the hair follicles and limits the medication's ability to fry the hair. It won't stop all the hair falling out, but it can help.' I read the leaflet, which stated that 60 per cent of patients have success with the scalp-cooling system. I decided to give it a shot and Riza brought in the machine. This was a bit more like it. It was about the size of an under-counter fridge crossed with an industrial hoover. Even better, it had an impressive elephant's-trunk tube coming from the mini freezer unit.

When Riza pulled the cap onto my head I thought I was going to expire from shock. It was like drinking a litre of Slush Puppie, coupled with the biggest snowball imaginable. When I say it was cold, it was Baltic. The snowball would stay in place for an hour prior to the chemotherapy and up to two hours after the dose had been administered.

'We need to make sure the drug doesn't have a chance to get at the scalp,' Riza explained. 'How does it feel?' She went down on her hunkers to speak to me. The machine made a dull hum, that was quite loud. My head, face, neck and shoulders were doused in clumps of ice. The pain through my skull was hideous. The actual bones felt like they were becoming rock solid – which I'm sure they were. I knew how it must feel to be a leg of lamb in the deep freeze. Can't say it was ever a personal yearning to have that information, but at least that box is ticked, should I ever wonder. I endured the cold for more than an hour. I was glad to be in a bed and pulled my covers up to my face.

They put a cannula, which is one of those needles with a bit of Lego attached to it, into a vein in my hand. The poison followed, one bag at a time, drip, drip, over a couple of hours. The entire dose, with flushes, took around four hours. A flush has nothing to do with a toilet. It's basically saline (a sterile salt-water solution) that is run through the drip in between each bag of drugs. It clears the lines and veins and makes sure that both are clean and ready to distribute or receive the next potion.

Hey presto, that was chemotherapy. Jaysus, I thought, I'm very good at this. I didn't feel sick at all.

My entire skull was in distress, though. My head felt like it had been on a school tour to the North Pole. My hair was white and crisp. I had the worst headache I'd ever experienced. I decided the cold cap was simply not worth the hassle. I'd tried and it was just too bloody cold. I hate being cold. It makes me ratty and I want to eat sweets. I didn't need to put on five stone while having chemotherapy. It was one thing doing that and producing a human being at the end of it, but I didn't think Cian would want to share a bed with a thawing baby hippo – even if it still had its own hair.

I can appreciate that anyone reading this might think, why on earth didn't she just get used to having a cold head every three weeks? And now that I write this, I nearly feel that way myself. But at the time I had the constant arthritis-style pain from the derma-tomyositis and, with the chemotherapy dumped on top, I simply couldn't cope with any more unpleasantness. The thought of losing my hair might have been enough to make me do anything to avoid it, but the decision to take my chances with alopecia seemed right for me at the time.

Most chemotherapy patients begin to feel the adverse effects a few days after each treatment. Due to my dermatomyositis, I experi-enced it differently. Dr Stafford had suspected the particular type of dermatomyositis I had came in conjunction with cancer, so the chemotherapy was multi-tasking. Not only was it blasting the shite out of the cancer, it was also killing the autoimmune disease. Marvellous stuff.

My treatments were administered at three-weekly intervals. So it took me two sessions before I began to notice any adverse reaction. Most patients notice the adverse effects a couple of days after the first session. But for me it took a bit longer. Seven weeks after I'd started, most of my hair had fallen out. It had become stringy and my scalp was becoming more and more visible. Although I felt very tired, the pain in my arms and legs from the autoimmune disease began to ease hugely. Contrary to what I had thought, the chemotherapy was actually making me feel better.

I came to the conclusion that I was a weirdo. I must have been the only person on the planet to feel better during chemotherapy. Maybe those women who told me they felt wonderful while they were pregnant weren't lying to belittle me and other women. Maybe it was possible to feel better, even when you're not supposed to.

It seems that most patients feel fine after the initial dose. It takes the chemotherapy a few days and often weeks to build up in the system. I know from chatting to other patients that the pattern appears to be this: if the chemotherapy is administered on Monday, by Thursday or Friday most people are feeling the effects. This typically means tiredness, nausea that can be mild or very severe depending on the patient (tablets help and it's worth trying a different one if the first or second doesn't work) and a general feeling of unease. It's worth noting that it's usual for this horrible crawly feeling and extreme tiredness to pass after one or two days.

As the treatments continue, the drugs build up in the system and the effects can become more pronounced. Once the dermatymyositis was arrested by the steroids, I too began to feel the adverse effects of the chemotherapy.

I found the best thing to do was balance my time between resting and doing things: I would make myself go to bed for an hour in the morning and again in the afternoon. Some days I felt like crawling under a rock and never coming out again. But I knew that that wasn't possible: I had a husband and two children. Also, it wasn't going to help me: even on the worst days, I knew the best policy was to haul my arse out of bed, stand under the shower and put on my clothes and make-up. Some of the time it was almost cruel, it caused me so much effort, but it was always worth it. I always felt better. Cutting myself off from everyone and everything never helped. Like those days when you've an awful hangover: it usually feels like a chore worse than execution to wash, dress and venture out in public, but even if it's just a trip to the local takeaway or a few minutes of fresh air, it can make all the difference. In my own little mind, I decided to treat the chemotherapy the same way. I decided it was a bad hangover. The only difference was the price: it was much cheaper than a night out, and I never needed something new to wear!

Chapter 23

No Hairs or Graces

A control freak? Who − me? You bet. Even when all the forces were telling me that I had no control, I grabbed the situation by the hair (pun very much intended) and soldiered on.

It was one of those balmy days when the sun was shining and instantly the world was a better place. My mum had just left the house with the children.

'Enjoy summer camp and I'll see you both later on. Don't forget to put on sun hats if you're outside like yesterday,' I'd reminded them.

'We won't. Bye, Mum,' Sacha said, hugging me. I knew they'd absolutely no intention of wearing their sun hats but it's always good, as a parent, to feel you've at least said the right thing − even if they totally ignore you.

I wasn't able to work at all at that point. My ability to move and do menial tasks, like the washing, had returned, however. The chemo-therapy and continued prednisolone had arrested the dermatomyositis. I had finished three sessions of chemotherapy and was settled back at home after spending an unbelievable seven weeks in hospital.

The chemotherapy had sapped every bit of energy I possessed. Perhaps it was due to the autoimmune disease too, but most of the time I felt like I'd been hit by a sledgehammer. Even the smallest exertion, like emptying the dishwasher, made me tired. I managed the children by organising camps and letting people take them to play, and Jane helped with cleaning and childminding and was another pair of hands.

As I went to step into the shower one morning towards the end of July, an entire section of my hair plopped onto my foot – the part just beside my ear, where I could see it. One minute it was on my head, the next it was on the bathroom floor. Not just a few strands, a handful. A clump. Enough to make a noise when it landed.

That was it. The hospital leaflets all gave the same advice on alopecia:

1. Don't shave your own head.
2. Don't look in a mirror while your hair is being removed. This may be too traumatic.
3. Don't go to the hairdresser alone. Bring a family member or supportive friend.
4. Prepare beforehand. Buy a wig or headscarf should you choose to cover your newly bald scalp.

So what did I do? None of the above. I grabbed Cian's hair clippers, stood in front of the bathroom mirror, in an empty house, and shaved every strand of my hair into the toilet.

How did I feel? Empowered.

If my hair was going to fry and fall out, then so be it: I couldn't stop it happening. By taking the clippers and shaving it myself, I felt in control. I rubbed my hand over my downy head. It felt soft and baby-like. I turned to the side. I was delighted to see I had a normal-shaped head. No big lumpy parts or uneven jutting-out bits. Not many people know whether or not they have a well-shaped head.

I hopped into the shower and was shocked by how hot the water felt on my hairless scalp. Drying myself afterwards was weird. I'd spent the weeks prior to this washing and brushing my hair as little as possible to preserve it. Also, as I'd always had fairly long hair, I automatically used two towels for a shower: a bath sheet and a smaller one to turban my dripping head.

When you have no hair, nothing drips. You dab your face dry, and that's it.

'Ha!' I said to the mirror. No wonder Cian had been shaving his head for so long. This was going to shave at least twenty minutes off each day – excuse the pun.

Then came a whole new problem. Dressing took ages. It took me half an hour to get dressed. None of my clothes went with baldness. That might sound utter tripe to you, but the style and colour of your hair can dictate a lot. When you've none, it's a real challenge.

The casual tracksuit style made me look like a gouger. I put on dressier clothes. That was worse: I looked like a drag queen. In jeans and a T-shirt, I looked like a baby boy. Dungarees would have been more fitting. I pulled on various hats, figuring that would cover it up. But we're used to seeing at least a few strands of hair protruding from a hat. Being shiny bald just looks odd. I resembled one of those kits we all had as children – where you buy a wooden spoon and there's a little pack with bobbly eyes, a round pom-pom for the nose and a smiley mouth.

By now, I was sweating and wanting to go out in my pyjamas and be done with it.

How was I supposed to put make-up on? My natural skin tone is milk bottle. With nausea and chemotherapy shading added to the mix, I wasn't attractive. I gained a whole new respect for Sinéad O'Connor. That girl is astonishingly beautiful: she can choose to be bald and still look better than most of us. I was glad I'd never taken the opportunity to flex my teenage tirade on my parents by shaving my head. Whatever about having to deal with this bald thing in my thirties, I would have looked a total fright as a gangly teenager.

My facial structure didn't look normal anyway. The steroids caused a horrible puffiness, so I didn't have gorgeous 'defined bone structure'. I was more along the lines of Mrs Play-Doh Face, when all the colours have got mixed in one pot and come out grey and nasty. The wig shop beckoned.

Knowing the children were safely running amok at camp, I called my mum.

'I look like a lollipop,' I moaned. 'We'll have to cut eyeholes in a black sack and find a wig shop pronto. This is not attractive, can you come now?'

As she came into my room, she gasped. Tears sprang forth. I didn't feel embarrassed, just dreadfully sorry to have had to make her look at me like that. This is the most appalling aspect of cancer in my experience. It's the devastation that is inflicted on the people closest to the patient. For me personally, I had, and still have, the inner strength to battle and fight. I never feel my own hope fading. Apart from the odd dark moment, I generally feel genuine positivity about my cancer. What I cannot control however is how my family and friends are going to feel as they witness what I'm going through. Putting myself in my parents' or husband's shoes, I feel immense guilt. I know I would hate to see my daughter lose her hair. It would break my heart. So in turn, I detest the fact that my darling mum had to deal with my baldness that day. The patient may have the internal fight and determination to protect them. Family and friends are the onlookers who would do anything in their power to help.

Mum has been amazing for the entire time since I first became ill. She ducks in and out of the house constantly, yet she never crowds me. Her calm and warm disposition had made her a wonderful Montessori teacher. That same soothing and easy nature was and still is a vital contribution to my battle with cancer. I never felt I couldn't tell her when I was feeling worried, scared, sad or, in this case, bald.

I can't imagine what she was going through. If the shoe was on the other foot and I had to watch her fighting cancer, I know I'd be useless. Whether or not it affected her, she never made that into my problem. She never buckled and she never made me feel like it was all too much for her. That day I had used the surge of inner strength that often grips me and had attempted to regain control of the fact that I was losing my hair. I had forced myself not to think of other people's reactions. I had simply concentrated all my efforts on doing the deed and shaving my head. I know I caused my mum to reel with shock when she saw me. I don't regret shaving my head but I hated upsetting my mum.

'Sorry, Mum, I know I look like a mutant baby. It had to go. We'll go and get hair now.' We hugged.

None of the people closest to me ever made me feel I was draining them. I had moments of darkness, when I felt racked with guilt and remorse, and wished that the cancer and the dermatomyositis would go away – not for myself: for my loved ones.

I wasn't happy looking like a bald baby, of course, and I didn't want my family and friends to see me with no hair. I know it's a totally personal choice and there's no right or wrong way to conduct yourself during cancer treatment, but I felt that if I wore a wig I might afford us all a few hours each day when we didn't have to be confronted with my cancer. For me, hiding my baldness was almost like time out from looking sick.

With my newly acquired baldness, I finally managed to choose some clothes to go wig shopping: I settled on a maxi-dress, which was long, flowing and pretty. It lent itself to the whole headscarf look.

Chapter 24

Not a Hair in the World

My trips to the hairdresser have been replaced by trips to the hair shop.

The first wig place Mum and I pitched up at was right up there with the electric chair in terms of comfort zones. 'It looks a bit dingy and depressing.' Mum screwed up her nose.

'Maybe it's one of those places that's really nice inside.' I tried to be upbeat.

We trundled into the shop, glancing back nervously, hoping the wheels would still be on the car when we came out. It wasn't the most affluent area of Dublin city.

The floors were covered in brown and cream lino. 'I haven't seen lino since the seventies. Now I remember why people don't buy it any more.' Mum shuddered.

The place smelt of budgie poo, and that wee-mixed-with-cabbage old-folks'-home stench.

'Yes?' An old buzzard appeared from nowhere, dressed in a nylon housecoat. She had a bristly chin and missing teeth.

'We're looking for a wig, and we found you in the *Golden Pages*,' I said, trying to be pleasant.

'Come and sit. I'll get May – we work better together,' said the buzzard.

'She could be male or female, but either way, she's bloody scary,' I whispered to Mum. The woman looked like a breeze block, with steel grey hair glued on badly by a small child. 'If she's offering hair like her own, I think I'll have to embrace the Kojak look.'

The beady-eyed budgie was clawing his way up the wall of his cage.

'Who's a pretty boy? Yes, you are.' The biddy made kissy noises at the bird, who reacted by squawking and headbanging.

May appeared. Like her partner, she was of the badger variety and only smiled at the budgie. I guessed I needed to have feathers and a Kelly-green tail to be afforded a smile.

'I'll bring you a selection and you can decide,' Buzzard Number One uttered, in a tight-lipped tone of annoyance.

'Lovely,' said Buzzard Number Two.

The first yoke they placed on my head must have been donated by the county council road-sweeping machine.

'No?' they chorused. They were emotionless either way about whether or not I loved their wigs.

Then, all of a sudden, it was like they kicked into action with a little play. One that the roadkill-wig manufacturers might have told them to do when they had to deal with cancer patients. Buzzard Number One kept patting my hand and doing a sort of watery-eyed, sniff-in-sympathy thing.

Now, before you yell that I'm a horrible cow, I'm sure some people like being treated like the living dead. They respond to the one-foot-in-the-grave mindset, but that's just not my buzz. I didn't want a lady in her seventies in a brown nylon cardigan yanking something that resembled a backcombed squirrel onto my bald head. Sorry, but I wasn't feeling the love.

Mum and I ran out of there, giggling and snorting like teenagers, and made our way to a city-centre store. There we met a girl who looked like a seventies punk, with a face so pierced she'd have blown up a metal detector. Unnecessarily loud music belted out of far too many speakers and the place smelt of glue.

'This is better,' Mum mouthed, and used sign language to communicate through the disco decibels.

'Hiya, I'm Lulu, whatcha after?' said the gum-chewing assistant, who had opted to dye her own hair lime-green.

'Hi, I've just shaved what was left of my hair and I don't want to look like a cancer victim,' I deadpanned.

'Cool. Follow me.' She seemed totally at ease with my situation and sauntered happily towards a little dressing table. She blew a bubble with her gum. 'Were you thinking long, short, curly, straight? And what colour? We have all sorts, so you tell me.'

'Well, I had straight blond hair before,' I ventured.

'Yeah, but that doesn't mean you have to look like that now. You can have bright pink curls if you like.' She grinned. 'Maybe get an everyday one and a fun one too.'

I tried on everything from Mohawks to Mary Quant bobs. Instead of feeling like we needed to go home and slit our wrists, Mum and I giggled with Lulu at some of the insane things she had on offer.

Aside from her wackiness, she had a good eye and knew what would suit me.

An hour later we left with two wigs, one long and one short, plus an array of scarves and hats.

'Stay cool, you'll be grand.' Lulu high-fived Mum and me and danced off to have a smoke out the back door of her shop.

Mum grinned. 'It's a bit ironic that she deals predominantly with cancer patients and she's obviously a chainsmoker!"

By the time we got home, we were wrecked. I put the bag of wigs on the hall table and we went into the kitchen for a cup of coffee and some sugar to soothe us. I began rooting in the usual hiding places for a secret stash of chocolate – not that any of them were secret any more: my children were as deft as circus performers at scaling cupboards and finding treasure.

They hadn't seen my lack of hair yet. I thought they might be frightened and astonished by my new look.

'Hi, Mum. Oh – you look just like Dad now. When did you shave your hair off?' Sacha asked. He tugged my sleeve. 'Bend down.' He stroked my head and smiled. 'Fuzzy.' He beamed up at me. 'Nice.' He seized the fleeting moment of weakness he'd cunningly spotted in my eyes and snatched a mini packet of Maltesers I'd unearthed from the pot cupboard under the cooker.

Kim skipped in. 'Oh, look, your hair is all gone. That's good – we got a letter from the summer-camp teacher about nits. Now you don't have to get the stinky stuff in your head.'

That was that. I said we'd have to get out the nit comb later, which sent them flying from the room. Anything to avoid the dreaded combing session.

I had bought a little soft T-shirt-material cap from Lulu, which she'd assured me would be handy for around the house. 'It'll stop you scaring the living daylights out of yourself every time you pass a mirror. Besides, it's bloody freezing having no hair.'

'Did you lose yours?' I asked. Maybe that was why she was in the wig business.

'Yes, love, but by choice. Bad dye job. It turned out a disgusting greyish-blue. I tried to fix it and I looked like a mangy grey squirrel, so I thought, sod it, and shaved the lot off. It's not like I'd be stuck for something to put on my head, is it?' She'd gestured around cheerfully.

As Mum and I tossed ideas around about an age-appropriate 'wig talk' with the children, we heard happy screeching emanating from the trampoline outside. Sacha had found one of my new wigs and put it on, back to front, with a pair of free-with-a-kid's-meal-at-Eddie Rocket's plastic sunglasses, and was chasing Kim. 'I am the hairy monster. I am going to eat your leg off, so you'd better keep away from me,' he was growling.

'Chat over and done with,' Mum remarked.

We took our drinks and went outside to pretend to be shocked by the scary monster.

I always wore a wig in public while I was bald. Believe me, there were days when I was on my hands and knees with exhaustion and sickness and felt like hiding under the duvet forever. But I would push myself to get up, have a shower and paint a smile on my face. Without fail, it helped. I understand it's a personal choice, but I never wanted to be a shining beacon, telling the world I was sick. I didn't want to be a cancer sufferer. I wanted to be a surfer. Fair enough, I would embrace the cancer thing, but I didn't need to publicise it with my bald head. Wearing my war paint and a wig allowed me to blend in. I could go to the supermarket or meet a friend for coffee, and people were none the wiser. It afforded me the chance to feel normal. It let me be the young woman I knew was inside the fug of sickness, drugs and cancer. I felt I was still me.

My qualification as a beauty therapist stood to me during that time. I could trowel on the make-up as well as any good plasterer – draw myself a mean set of eyebrows and literally paint on some healthy skin. In the seventies, it was impossible to wear too much Virgin Mary-blue eye shadow. When you're going through chemotherapy, apply that same notion with bronzer. Trust me, it works. A normal complexion ends up looking orange; a chemo patient looks almost normal.

There are programmes called 'Look Good, Feel Better' running worldwide. They do exactly what their title suggests and it's free to patients. They are well worth checking out.

I also used fake tan. I'm a fan of the tan anyway, but while I was sick it was essential. Due to the rash, which was thankfully fading, my complexion was mottled – it looked like that scary pink-veined cheese. You know the one – it looks like Stilton made by a colour-blind toddler? That was my face and body. Not attractive.

I asked Dr Fennelly if I was allowed to use tanning products. His thoughts on it were that any confidence and happiness you can muster up during treatment is worth a shot. There is a school of thought that bans the use of chemicals and additives forever should you have a cancer diagnosis, but as I've already said, I do that in moderation. For me, make-up and a sense that I didn't look as if I'd been dug up after a night of grave-robbing meant a lot. I will give you some suggestions of brands that I find effective at the end of the book.

Shopping is another great thing. Retail therapy works. Trust me. I don't mean you have to go to Harvey Nicks and spend two grand on a ball gown (although I would applaud you if you did!). A trip to Primark or Topshop to buy a pair of socks, or into Boots for a lipstick, can be a brilliant pick-me-up.

Never underestimate the power of chocolate. I know chemotherapy causes some very weird taste changes, but good quality chocolate is always a winner. If crisps are your thing, buy the really nice black-pepper ones. If jellies are your buzz, get a large bucket of Jelly Bellys. Basically, be nice to yourself. You've enough nasty stuff to deal with, so a little treat goes a long way. You're worth it, as the L'Oréal people say.

Another side effect of my chemotherapy was ridges on my nails – as if someone had drawn across the nail bed with a Tipp-Ex pen.

They became fairly noticeable, as my nails tend to grow quite long. In spite of all my sickness, I always seem to have strong nails. I didn't have a huge problem with this, and if I had the energy to go anywhere at night, I would lash on a coat of polish. But I did meet several women in my hospital travels who were quite bothered by this. There's a wonderful product that Tesco sells. It's a clear nail polish, which can be used as a topcoat or by itself. It's called Goodbye Yellow. It has a slight ultraviolet effect and makes stained or marked nails look whiter and healthier. There are lots of expensive ones that do the same or perhaps an even better job, but that one worked for me. I am a slave to Shellac these days. I can do it myself but more often than not I pop to my local nail bar where I can have a full manicure and Shellac done for 20 euros – I think it's worth every cent and it lasts for at least two weeks.

Clarins do a cult product called *Beauty Balm*. Well worth a purchase! You can apply it under make-up or on its own (if you have better skin than me). Again, it helps with the deathly pallor and gives the impression of a glow. I don't work for any of these companies: their products are just little bits and bobs I found along the way. Sadly, there aren't any money-off coupons for them at the back of this book! And if any of the cosmetics houses feel the need to send me an enormous box of nice stuff, I promise to share.

I didn't wallow in the negative aspects of my illness. I didn't accept that I would stay sick indefinitely. I always had faith in my health carers and myself, and that this was merely transient. It was not a permanent fixture. Even now, ten years on, I have hope that some day science will help me beat cancer for good.

We all have bad days. Of course I do too – I wouldn't be human if I didn't. In September 2007, I was at an all-time low. I'd been suffering constant infections. I'd been stabbed to within an inch of my life by phlebotomists (these are the people who are specifically trained to take blood). I love them all dearly and they know I call their actions 'stabbing'! I was, in a word, shipwrecked.

'I'm broken,' I sighed to my friend. 'I'm actually considering clubbing myself over the head and getting it over with in a more humane manner. Maybe they could boil my skin off and make me into a nice coat or something.'

Cathy Kelly, my guardian angel on earth, decided we should go to Monart for a night. This place is marketed as a spa. I don't think that's a good enough word for what it does. It's a sanctuary for restoring sanity, in my humble experience. Others may not share my view, but that was how I found it.

We dumped our bags in our room, a tranquil, soothing space full of squashy calm. It was a bit like being in a pot of clotted cream. We had driven there, which meant we'd filled Cathy's entire boot and back seat with everything from walking gear to six changes of clothes.

After an hour in the place, before we'd even had any treatments, we already felt more relaxed. All the warmth, the yards of thick carpet, the swishy music and the lack of any need to think are just divine. In fact, it should be mandatory for us all to go somewhere like that once a week – Fridays should become pyjama days for everyone.

Most people were having some sort of face and body petting, so we thought we'd better do the same. Everyone had greasy hair, slicked back with essential oils, and slightly peeled-looking features. I thought it would be a bit cringy, and we'd be asking for masks so we didn't look a sight. But it just didn't matter.

They encouraged long walks through their Fairyland landscape – they even provided wellies and umbrellas – but it was lashing rain, so Cathy and I settled for a quick dash outside along a pretty moss-surrounded path to the steaming shed. I'm sure it has a romantic Swedish name but it was basically a posh garden shed that worked like a people-sized bamboo steamer. Instead of cooking a field of cabbage all at the same time, they were using it for cooking toxins out of people. There are lots of different people-ovens in the place. You can start in gentle wafty heat and work your way up to pressure-cooking yourself, should you so wish.

If you're having too much fun and are relaxing so much you're in danger of becoming incontinent or losing the power of your legs, you're welcome to give yourself near heart failure with a plunge pool or cold shower. I myself don't understand the ice-cold, shock-the-shite-out-of-yourself way of thinking. I prefer to loll on a bench, go with the hot flushes and embrace the purple, head-like-a-turnip look. It passes after a few minutes. Besides, a glass of water, once you've stopped hallucinating and having vertigo from overheating, works wonders.

I had a head massage, which made me lose all power in my entire body and dribble. Not attractive for the poor therapist, to have a drooling creature on her couch, but lovely for me. We finished by having our paws petted and nails painted.

We'd agreed to wait for each other before going back to the room. As Cathy approached, I decided I'd better sit for a second. I'd been upright for over five minutes by that point. We ended up beside each other on yet another nest of comfy sofas. We had an enlightening monosyllabic in-depth conversation.

'Nice?'

'Um.'

'You?'

'Um.'

'Better?'

'Um.'

'You?'

'Um.'

They almost had to remove us by forklift truck the next afternoon. We were brave and didn't whinge or try to hold on to the door knocker as they helped us put the unworn contents of our houses back into Cathy's car.

I know it's not always feasible to go to a spa or even a hotel for a break. But if it's within your grasp, do it. It would be worth selling your kitchen table and chairs or the living-room furniture on eBay to do this. Have a go at the type of stuff they do on that show on television where they scan the entire house for things that you don't necessarily use and sell them. Or find a friend who lives a little bit away from your own house and beg a spare bed for the night. The change of scene and not having to cook are a breath of fresh air.

I can't stress enough how amazing it is for your mind and body to be pampered and allowed to unwind. It's worth its weight in gold.

Chapter 25

Stab City

A qualification as an overnight nurse. Marvellous. Did I miss my calling in life? Was I supposed to have been a junkie? Is it normal to feel this excited about injecting myself?

By October 2007, I was five months into my treatment. As my chemotherapy continued, I learned lots of new and impressive words. By the time my cancer diagnosis had come through, I could already hold my own, talking nonchalantly about a bilateral prophylactic mastectomy and oophorectomy. While I sipped a cold glass of Chardonnay, I could happily discuss post-surgical pain management. But now, since I'd joined the chemo club, I knew all about neutropenia too.

No, it's not a sexually transmitted disease. Neither is it a little-known island off Africa, nor a grungy pop group comprising long-haired young men with bad attitudes and a penchant for Captain Morgan's rum. It's when your neutrophils are low – in other words, when the chemotherapy has zapped the hell out of your system and you've no white blood cells. The white cells help to fight infection. One of the side effects of chemotherapy is that these little cells are destroyed.

All oncology patients will be familiar with the 'Phil' poster campaign. Phil is a blue superhero character. He's like Superman, but he's entirely electric blue for some reason. He has a cape, very defined muscles, wears his underpants over his trousers and stands in a Mr Universe pose, with a cheesy grin. Being entirely blue, he's more like someone from *Avatar* than a medical hero, but he is the guy you want in your life. All the posters are set out in a pre school manner. The writing is big and clear: 'Do you know about Phil?' It goes on to tell us how to look after Phil and what to do if he's low. Sadly it doesn't involve bringing Phil to Monart or down the pub for a few pints. Instead, the poster insists you have a blood test and get your health carer to monitor your neutrophils.

'What do you do if Phil is low?' The answer to this one isn't great either. It doesn't involve buying a Prada handbag or a nice pair of Wolford tights. Instead you have a little list of danger signs:

1. Any temperature over 38°C indicates fever.
2. Shaking chills.
3. Sore throat.
4. Cough or shortness of breath.
5. Nasal congestion.
6. Diarrhoea or loose bowels.
7. Burning during urination.

Needless to say, like all chemotherapy patients, I became obsessed with my temperature. I bought one of the little hand-held digital thermometers, which I brought everywhere in my handbag. In the beginning, in my innocence, I thought I'd have to keep checking for signs of fever. I became a bit of an obsessive-compulsive, producing the device and poking it into my ear, then waiting for the beep.

I naïvely assumed I would have to be certain to the exact degree whether or not I was febrile. It was a little bit like my first pregnancy, when I asked the genuinely innocent question: 'But how will I know I'm in labour?' Ha! Just like the first time I went into labour, all the thermometer fixation changed after the first time I got an infection. There was no wondering involved. It was like I'd swallowed an industrial heater. My eyeballs were vibrating from side to side and my teeth were chattering like I'd been left in a deep freeze overnight.

I did use my thermometer (obsession is obsession, fever or not) and instead of the usual 37.0°C or even 36.8°C that my temperature had been until now, it read 38.8°C. This was a full-scale red alert. If

I'd owned a helmet with a flashing light and bee-baw siren, it would've come into use.

I rang the hospital and reported the thermometer reading, involuntary eye movement and chattering of teeth.

'Come straight in,' said the oncology nurse.

That meant 'immediately'. Do not go to Tesco or Dundrum shopping centre on the way. Do not pass go, do not collect €200.

The drill that followed at Blackrock Clinic was administered with military precision. A blood sample was taken. Blood pressure, temperature and all vital signs were checked. They asked half a phone book's worth of questions, and a drip was inserted before I could blink. The same cannot be said of other establishments. I'll tell you about that later.

During chemotherapy, they do what's called a routine mid-cycle blood test. This is between treatments, and they check to see what your white cells (our pals, the neutrophils), red cells and platelets are up to. The red cells are for carrying oxygen around the body. The platelets are for coagulating – so if you cut yourself, you don't bleed to death. All very handy. All very necessary.

Due to my added bonus of the autoimmune disease, I nearly always ended up with a grand total of zero white cells. Nada. I never knew it was possible to fail a blood test, but there you have it: I'm quite talented when it comes to sickness.

But all was not lost. The clever little fairies in the oncology profession had an answer to everything. 'Fear not,' they cried, 'you shall have Neupogen injections.' This magic stuff basically runs straight to the bone marrow and stimulates it to create more infection-fighting white fellas. Bloody brilliant! Whoever invented that was a genius. There are two types of these injections. One is called Neulasta, which is given once per chemotherapy cycle. The other is Neupogen, which is given daily for up to ten days. Neulasta is a slow-release version, and Neupogen is a progressive build-up version.

I discovered through trial and error that Neupogen would work better for me. This part was beyond exciting. I got to take home a tiny little mouse's version of the big yellow sharps buckets that hospitals have. God, I was so impressed. It was like being a nurse, just like that, without having to go to college or do work experience wiping old people's arses. I was beside myself. In fact, the yellow vessel was only the beginning. I got a whole going-home bag of party stuff to play nurses with.

'I can tell by the look on your face that you're not too fazed by having to do injections.' Mechelle smiled.

'This is the best fun ever. Look at all the stuff!' I clapped my hands in glee.

'Emma, you're not meant to be that thrilled by the prospect of injecting yourself.'

Perhaps I was a heroin addict in a former life. The idea of having my very own, let's pretend hospital kit was a buzz.

'OK, along with the antiseptic swabs and the fun-size sharps bucket, you'll need these.' Mechelle showed me the *pièce de résistance* of the entire game. Fully loaded and ready-to-stab hypodermics!

'Ooh! I'm impressed, now my fridge can look just like a vet's practice.'

From that day on, beside the milk and the leftover baked beans from the night before, there was a pile of slim cardboard boxes.

'Now you need to watch, listen and learn. If you feel in any way freaked, we can organise an oncology nurse to come to your house,' Mechelle promised.

'Are you joking? This is my chance to be a nurse and play hospital. Unless I'm in danger of stabbing myself to death or ending up jerking around in a circle, biting my own tongue in two, I want this gig,' I assured her.

'OK, I hear you loud and clear. You're scaring me a little. It's not supposed to be uproariously exciting.' She giggled.

'I'm an oddball. Work with me here.' We couldn't stop cackling.

'Every day, at the same time, give yourself an injection. If you think of it, take the shot out of the fridge half an hour before you administer the dose.'

'Why? Will it not work as well otherwise?'

'No, nothing like that, it'll just feel really cold. If it's nearer to room temperature, it'll be less unpleasant,' she explained.

Mechelle put on disposable gloves and opened a little packet, like the ones you get for wiping your hands on a plane. 'So, sit on a chair, swab the area, pat dry with a clean piece of cotton wool, pinch up some tummy flab …'

'Not that you're suggesting that I or any other patient would actually own tummy flab,' I added helpfully.

'Of course.' Mechelle didn't miss a beat. 'When you've managed to locate some flesh, insert the needle at 90 degrees. Press down gently to release the Neupogen. Then dispose of the used needle in the yellow sharps bin.'

'So will I try one now, then?' I was like a child with her face pressed against the oven waiting for the cookies to bake.

'Go for it.'

It all went swimmingly at the hospital. I was all business and even tried to pretend I was calm for a split second. Then I broke cover and leaped around like a mad thing, shouting that I'd done my first ever injection.

Once I'd started injecting at home, the rules and orderly calm didn't always prevail. If I'm honest, it usually involved both children and the cat. Kim became obsessed with wanting to join in. I would let her swab my tummy, and Sacha could open the box. They'd both gasp, immeasurably impressed that we had injections in our house.

All kids that came on a play date around that time were introduced to our syringes in the fridge. This is another reason why it can be good to level with people when you are sick. How else would I have stopped my children being taken into care when their friends told their parents they'd been looking at Emma's needles?

The downside of the Neupogen injections was a tummy full of mini bruises, like an elderly banana, and the bone pain. Because the medication stimulates the bone marrow, it causes any areas of bone density, such as pelvis, hips, knees and ankles, to ache. By day ten of the injections, I'd get mad, random shooting pains. I'd be strolling in the supermarket or meandering down the road and bam, a vicious shot, followed by another, then two more. It was damn difficult not to look as if I was being attacked by an invisible man, stabbing me in the lower back.

Although I can't say it was enjoyable to experience this kind of pain, the voice of reason whispered, 'Embrace that shooting pain, Emma. It's doing its job. It's inviting Phil and his blue superhero buddies into your bone marrow. They'll have a massive party and make white blood cells all night.'

There is such a thing as constructive pain.

'Are you getting dead, Mummy?' Sacha asked one night, during that time.

'No, love. I'm doing the opposite.'

'But you're in bed a lot. You can't bounce on the trampoline any more. Why? Does the cancer hurt a lot?' he asked.

'No, the cancer doesn't hurt at all. It's the medicine that's making me sick. Do you know why?'

'No.' He crossed his legs and stared at me.

'It's really busy, running around my blood and using its tiny gun to kill all the bad cells. They're the cancer guys. They run all the time, and it makes my blood and my body so tired. But at the end of it, the bad guys will all be dead, and I'll be able to bounce again. OK?'

'Will that be tomorrow?' He cocked his head to the side.

'No, not until just before Santa comes. But once Santa's been, we'll all feel better.'

'Why can't the hospital give you a different medicine? One that doesn't make you so tired. Do they know it does that?' Sacha asked.

'Yes, they know, and they're very sorry about it, but every time I go into the hospital and they give me more medicine, the cancer gets killed a little bit more.'

'I think you should pretend you went in and just stay at home. That way you'll be able to go to the cinema and bowling tomorrow,' he figured.

'It doesn't work that way, honey. This is the only medicine they know of that kills my type of cancer. The doctors and nurses know that it makes me, and the other people who have cancer, tired. They're really kind to me and they always give me scones and coffee. But they've promised me I won't feel like this for that much longer. None of this is forever. It's only for a while. After the tiredness goes away I'll be all better. So it'll be worth it in the end.'

'That's good, Mum. You just rest and maybe you should keep going to get that medicine. Do they have bars of chocolate in there too?'

'Yes – I can go to the shop you've been into. I'm allowed to walk around and get things if I feel like it.'

The staff at The Blackrock Clinic were amazing with Sacha and Kim. I told the nurses about Sacha's questions, and they immediately told me I could bring them in with me next time I was having a blood test. It worked brilliantly. Kim was given a nurse's badge – Sacha didn't want one – and they were allowed to sit in the big leather chairs in the Oncology day unit. I showed them the drip stands; they rooted in the fridge and stole some biscuits.

'OK, let's go and see the vampire lady in here,' I joked.

Helen and Kinjal were my lovely stabbers at the time. How they smile every day while working with needles is beyond me.

'Let's see if we can make Mum's blood jump from inside her body into a little bottle,' Helen said.

'Does it hurt when the needle goes in your blue thing?' Kim stood with her face right up against mine.

'It pinches for a second, and then it's fine.'

Both children loved the phlebotomists' trolley, with all the plasters and implements.

'Now here comes Mummy's blood into the special bottle. Then we'll put a sticker on it so everyone knows it belongs to her.'

'In case someone thinks it's from a cat or dog?' Kim wondered.

'Well, more in case they think it belongs to another person.' Helen kept a straight face.

The trip in for a blood test was short but the kids were able to see exactly where I was going every few weeks and had a visual image of what was happening to me.

'So isn't it great in here?' I said cheerfully. 'Will we say goodbye to the nurses now?'

'Bye, Sacha, bye Kim,' they all chorused.

'They even know our names. It's a bit like we're famous, isn't it?' Kim giggled.

The thing that astonished me most about Sacha and Kim was how little they noticed my appearance. They knew I wasn't up trees or doing as much baking, and commented from time to time. But when I was bald, the colour of putty and barely able to move with exhaustion, they would launch themselves at me and hug me, babbling about their day at school. They didn't seem to see the distorted version of Mum. They didn't scrutinise or seem to notice the same things that I saw when I looked in the mirror. They simply saw Mum. Just the way she always was. For that unconditional love and devotion, I will be eternally grateful.

Cian was amazing too. When we got married, we wanted to be together, of course we did. We said 'for better, for worse, in sickness and in health'. But we were twenty-five and twenty-four respectively. I know we were old enough to appreciate what we were getting ourselves into, but saying and doing are two very different things. If ever there was a time when our love and marriage were tested, it was while I was ill. Neither of us had signed up for what was thrown at us. How would Cian have responded if the priest at our wedding had said, in that mumbly eyes-half-shut way:

'Will you stand by this woman while she has half her body chopped off? She will have cancer ten times. She'll look like a boiled chipmunk and won't be able to stay awake past nine o'clock at night for three years. Will you?'

I don't think the most impressive couture wedding gown, the promise of €1 million a year in compensation to spend on racing bikes and a customised Porsche would have made any sane man say, 'I will.'

But Cian stayed. He supported me, loved me and made me laugh: 'Jesus, you look rough. Could you not have made a bit more effort, knowing I was going to drop in?' he mocked, as he bent to kiss me one morning when he arrived in the hospital. I was incarcerated with yet another infection. During those awful times, there were no words that fitted. Saying 'you look great' would have resulted in his having a set of nail clippers embedded in his forehead. I don't do fibs and I hate insincerity. But having someone who could make me laugh, and laugh along with me, was what held us together.

Some women need a bouquet of flowers each week. They expect heart-shaped boxes of chocolates and gushy cards on Valentine's Day. If their diamonds aren't bigger than everyone else's in the car park at school, they go into a dark hole of depression. With all my hospital visits, I have had more flowers than the most popular grave in the cemetery. I buy my own chocolate – I don't see it as a treat: it's a food group.

I think Valentine's Day is a sack of shit. Cian buys Sacha chocolates and Kim flowers on 14 February. They both grin for a week. But we don't do the overpriced meal and feeling like a goon amongst eighty other tables for two. I like diamonds, and would never refuse one (for the record), but they are not the meaning of love for me.

I know the meaning of love. He's still here. He's never wavered. He's never made me feel any less of a woman than I was the day we met. That to me is utterly priceless. I am also aware of how fortunate I am to have my teenagers and my husband still by my side.

From what I've been told, age makes all the difference with fertility and chemotherapy. Women in their twenties and thirties seem to be able to tolerate higher doses of chemotherapy for longer periods and still maintain fertility. Some women can lose fertility for a short time, and regain it once the chemotherapy is behind them. Radiation can also cause infertility, depending on the area being treated. For example, if the radiation is being carried out extensively on the pelvic region, it can adversely affect the ovaries or testicles.

Some doctors offer egg retrieval as an option. If the eggs are fertilised and frozen as embryos, they can be implanted later and result in healthy pregnancy. But each case is different, depending on the length of time available to the patient.

I will never take my children for granted. Not a day passes that I don't thank my lucky stars they are mine, In spite of the fact that they are teenagers and most of what I do is wrong!

Chapter 26

Dr Emma at Your Service

If you have an ill — I have a pill. Come on over to my place!

Before I got sick, a person with a hangover or headache would have been in dire straits in our house. I never had so much as a paracetamol in the cupboard. In fact, I attached a strong sense of guilt to pain-killers or any medication at all. Perhaps it's an Irish thing, or maybe it's more Austrian. Oma, my maternal grandmother, was a great woman for saying, 'It's not life threatening,' when we were growing up.

My parents were always very kind and sympathetic when we were children — don't think for a second that they weren't — but we never had plasters, creams, potions or much medicine in the house. If you fell, you got dabbed with a bit of Dettol, which stung the leg off you. For all other ailments it was either two Disprin or a big spoon of Milk of Magnesia. It wasn't really worth having anything too wrong: the cure was so vile it didn't encourage complaining!

Since my children have come along, the incentive to be ill is so much greater. Calpol and kids' Nurofen taste like melted jelly sweets. Plasters have everything from Disney characters to Justin Bieber's face on them. Doctors' waiting rooms are expected to have in-house entertainment. Being sick is much more fun these days.

My house, pre-cancer, was like Old Mother Hubbard's when it came to drugs. I actually remember rooting in a cupboard to find something to help a friend with a dreadful hangover. 'You have to have Solpadeine or Panadol, for the love of God. What do you do if you're in agony?' She flopped onto the kitchen table, smelling of stale vodka.

'I really don't have anything bar Sudocrem, bite spray, which is two years out of date, a dried-up bottle of Gaviscon from my pregnancy and a small bottle of Calpol from Sacha's MMR injections last month,' I apologised.

'Jesus, you're useless. Give me the Calpol. That has paracetamol, hasn't it?' She looked suitably unimpressed.

'It does, but it's really sticky and sweet. Are you sure you'll hold it down?' I worried.

'My head is separating – it can't make me any worse,' she moaned.

It was quite successful, as it turned out. It was so sweet it made her vomit violently – she narrowly made it to the bathroom. Her hangover was much better afterwards. She was so traumatised after the impromptu puking that her head forgot to ache. So, results all around.

Now, however, post-cancer, our house is like a pharmacy. I have dubbed myself Dr Emma. I have everything from full courses of antibiotics to class 'A' painkillers, sleeping tablets and an entire range of stomach-lining pills. I had a brief problem accepting the amount of pharmaceuticals I was having to take. I really felt like I should rattle when I walked. But the main point was this: all the things I was using were making me well. The cancer was going away. When I got infection after infection during chemotherapy, the antibiotics killed it.

Many people are against Western medicine, preferring to use alternative things. I respect that. I tried it. It nearly killed me. I won't do it again.

I am sensible with my diet. I understand food and know how to cook it. I eat fresh ingredients, organic meat and I rarely drink. I do love chocolate, but I only eat enough to satisfy my daily craving. I have come to terms with that addiction. I am at peace with and take full personal responsibility for my chocoholism.

I also bought a juice masticator. You must pronounce that word correctly or it might be in danger of sounding obscene. Mum was the juicer in our houses. She had the patience to grind fruits and vegetables and make wheatgrass shots for us all to gag on. Wheatgrass is meant to have all sorts of magic powers. It's supposed to be the

Rolls-Royce of fuel to boost our entire system. I did drink it for a while but I found it utterly vile and I can't even pretend it did me any good. In fact, it was so disgusting that I felt virtuous after downing a shot of it. It's in the category of stuff that's so awful, it must be good for you.

I know there are many healthy people who will say I'm being ridiculous and that wheatgrass is actually quite nice. That I should love the earthy taste of raw beetroot and carrot juice – indeed, I can add a dash of honey to make it taste really delicious. Sorry, I can't pretend it's yummy. I equate it to licking the spoon after feeding the cat. It's just not my buzz – but I'm a heathen and believe the world would be a better place if Xanax or Valium was put in the general water supply and we all ate chocolate for breakfast. I know I'm a bad, bad person and probably sending out the wrong vibe. But I can't help how I feel. I have moved on to smoothies using a NutriBullet. I go for fruits and seeds and almond milk and make drinks that are more like a McDonald's milkshake than sludge from the bottom of a pond. The upside of using fruits and berries is that the teenagers will take them too.

In my defence, I'm not entirely bad. I don't think I should be expelled from healthy school altogether. I eat porridge every morning, with birdseed and soya yoghurt on it. The birdseed is a mixture of goji berries, flax seeds, sunflower seeds and other pet-shop fodder. That's pretty impressive, isn't it? I also force myself to glug down as many pints of water as possible each day. Again, it's a habit I have to make myself continue. I stand at the sink and, using my filter tap, (because the water is meant to be better for me), brace myself and drink it as quickly as I can. Anyone looking in the window would be forgiven for thinking I was lowering a pint of vodka. I'm just not a fan of water. It makes me screw my face up and shudder. I don't eat wheat as it bloats me and works like a cork for my bowels.

The oncology team are obsessed with bowels and whether or not they're moving. Wheat is obviously like a stun gun for my bowels. Not only do they refrain from moving, but they seem to decide they are a storage unit. From what I can make out, chemotherapy does one of two things to them. Either you shit through the eye of a needle and become skeletal. Or, like me, you have a magic skip for a bowel that has a 50 litre capacity. Believe me it's not a good sensation to carry a week of food around in your innards. The entire time I am on chemotherapy, I use two things, Movicol (which is prescription only) and Senokot. It's a senna-based laxative, which is meant to help the bowel move in a gentle way. In the end I had to ask the hospital to put them on prescription for me. If I tried to buy Senokot in any pharmacy bar my local one, where they all know me, I'd get the look.

I wasn't overweight, so people would assume that I was planning on eating laxative sandwiches, washed down with castor-oil smoothies. 'Can I have a box of twenty-four Senokot, please?'

On more than one occasion, I got the arms folded below the bosom, and the austere look.

'The most I'll sell you is twelve,' one particularly narky assistant spat, looking me up and down.

'It's not what you think. I'm having chemotherapy, and the side effect for me is severe constipation. I'm taking them under strict medical supervision,' I assured her.

'Yes, of course you are.' She smirked.

I know it was bold. I know I should have taken a deep breath and risen above the situation. I should have seen it from her point of view and accepted the smaller packet, knowing I would go to my local pharmacist in a few days. But I wasn't having a charitable-attitude moment.

I had just finished a grocery shop. The cupboards were so bare it looked like we'd just moved in. I'd yelped when the girl at the till had told me what I owed. But I knew I'd replenished everything from jam and ketchup to meat and fruit. It was lashing rain, my feet were freezing and I'd had no coffee yet.

In the chemist's, I pulled my wig off and stood, nostrils flaring, with eyes like a murderer. 'Now do you believe me?'

'Oh, em, sorry. I didn't know—'

'No, you didn't, did you? But I tried to tell you and you had just made up your mind. Next time you decide to jump to the wrong conclusion and stand with that smug, know-it-all expression, think again.'

I yanked my wig on sideways and marched out of the shop. Needless to say, I have never set foot in that pharmacy again and I will use my bare hands to dig a trench should I ever see that woman approaching me in the street.

I know I'm prone to the odd outburst, but I try to be good in other ways. I don't drink beer or spirits; it's months since I've had any alcohol as I simply haven't been able to drink. But when I do – I just stick to red wine or champagne. Not because I'm a martyr, but because that's what I like.

I use fake tan and make-up. I use shower gel and body lotion. I know it's probably tested on racoons and some believe they are all carcinogenic. But I feel I have to have a quality of life. If I had to go around with no make-up on, I would end up in a straitjacket – which would make scratching rather difficult.

I asked Dr Fennelly if I had to wear knitted shoes and eat only leaves and drink water from waterfalls out of a unicorn horn. Thankfully he told me to be sensible. If I'm eating fresh, healthy food, and taking regular exercise, that's the key. Everything in moderation. There is no clinical evidence that wearing make-up causes cancer.

In truth I do look on the labels of beauty products too. Just to make sure they don't contain parabens. My skin care range is all Clarins as it is plant based and free of nasties. But there are a whole host of products on the market now that are paraben free. The key is to find one that suits. Ask at the cosmetic counters for samples and you'll know which one suits your skin.

Cian is a triathlon bunny. He is obsessed with swimming, running and cycling. He gets a buzz out of all this body beating. He and his fellow triathlon lunatics discuss times, transitions and optimising training. I am as lazy as sin. I hate exercise. There, I said it. The only reasons I do any, are: (a) so my heart and body don't go kaput; (b) so my thighs don't end up the size of China.

I think each one of us has to do what suits us. I know there are many people who feel the alternative medicine route works for them. That homeopathy and herbal medicine are the way to go. Many believe that Western doctors shouldn't pump cancer patients with toxic drugs. I respect that, but I'm terrified by the lack of legislation governing alternative practitioners. For me, Western medicine and my oncology team have worked. I am still here. I am still alive. That is all the proof I need that I am doing what works for me.

Chapter 27

Promotion!

I am on my way up the chemotherapy ladder. I get to become a 'day case' rather than an 'in-patient'. I'm oddly nervous. Will the Oncology unit be like a den of despair? Will it be heaving with semi-dead skeletal reptiles, all of whom used to resemble humans?

By my fifth session of chemotherapy, the dermatomyositis had improved enough that I was promoted to the Oncology day unit. I had been at home since my previous treatment and had managed a full two weeks without seeing the inside of the hospital. My energy levels were still very low. There was no question of being able to work or even spend a day walking around the shops. I had to balance my rest time with my up-and-about time.

For me, that bout of chemotherapy was like a job in itself. It was all-consuming, exhausting, and I had to fit my life around it. The only difference between the treatment and a job was the method of payment. In a real job you get a pay packet at the end of the week or month. At the end of the chemotherapy, I was hoping to get my life back. So although my bank balance mightn't have gained much during that time, my work was going to enrich me in the most important way possible.

My progression to the Oncology day unit was the best promotion I could seek during my chemotherapy job. It meant I was allowed to go in on the morning of treatment and return home that afternoon. Prior to this I had been so sick, I'd had to go into hospital and stay overnight so that the medical staff could monitor me for twenty-four hours.

'You won't be having any more sleepovers in Hotel Blackrock?' Kim mused.

'Not for the moment, I hope. I'll just go in and have the chemo-therapy medicine and come back here.'

I didn't want to say I'd never go back for a sleepover, just in case I was taken in with an infection. The one thing I had learned was that children are like elephants – not large, grey and wrinkly, but they never forget. No matter what was thrown at me, I didn't want to lie to mine or keep them in the dark. I learned to work with the facts. Once they were put in the picture on a regular basis, Sacha and Kim seemed to be satisfied. Now ten years later, they are in their late teens and we can have open, more adult discussions about cancer. Thankfully, they are never afraid to ask questions.

I was actually nervous the first time I stood in the day unit. I had a sense of foreboding. Would I be greeted by a stench of dying people and a fug of illness that would chill me to the bone? Would it be full of people writhing in pain and climbing the walls, begging God to put them out of their misery?

As it turned out, the day unit was a large bright room with spacious areas and windows. There were eight big chairs – four against each wall, separated in the centre by a coffee-and-tea-making facility – and a bathroom. The chairs were those very plush, and no doubt expensive, leather recliner ones, with the ability to shunt backwards so a footrest shoots out, should you want to lie back.

Two private consultation rooms were available for patients to talk to a doctor or nurse in peace. The people occupying the chairs all looked totally normal. If they were bald, none of them looked it. It was wigs or natural hair all the way. There was a mixture of age groups, although none seemed younger than me. The atmosphere was relaxed and friendly. One person was reading a newspaper, another a book. A man was making himself a cup of coffee and cutting up a scone.

'Hi, Emma, I'm Lisa, one of the oncology nurses. Pick a chair and I'll be with you in a jiffy.'

I found an empty seat and perched on the edge. For a few moments,

I simply looked around. There were drip stands behind each chair, but aside from that, it wasn't an outlandishly weird environment. Some people chatted – they recognised each other from previous days. Others listened to iPods. Within half an hour I felt at ease. There was no air of death. Nobody crawled on the floor creating a trail of vomit. Nobody was coughing up blood or being held down and tortured. It didn't even seem to be compulsory to attempt to pretend you were on the way out. Not a retch or a groan in earshot.

I got up, ventured towards the kitchenette area, made myself some coffee and helped myself to a bottle of chilled water. Within minutes, I was shown into one of the side rooms. The usual questions were asked, ranging from how I was feeling, to how I was sleeping, to the inevitable bowel-movements question. Hospitals are obsessed with stools and the frequency of them. Next, I was passed to the phlebotomy room, where they took blood and put in a cannula. Just the same as the other times in my room, the bags of chemotherapy were administered one by one. By four o'clock I was ready to drive home.

My chemotherapy was supposed to be completed within six months. It ended up taking seven. As Phil was absent without leave (maybe he had secured a job as an extra on *Avatar*), I had no white blood cells, in spite of the injections. I ended up with pneumonia, urinary-tract infections, chest infections and, more than once, a mystery illness that caused a hideously high temperature and general sickness. The medics put these under the umbrella of 'neutropenic infections'. The body is in serious danger of not being able to fight off the infection and get well, so it means a hospital stay each time. Discharge is only allowed when the patient has been free of fever for more than twenty-four hours.

Each time an infection hit, I had to have intravenous antibiotics, stay in hospital for up to a week and push back my chemotherapy until I was strong enough to take it. Not happy with delaying everything and ending up back as an inmate in the hospital, I decided to frighten the living daylights out of Mechelle.

Mechelle was one of the oncology nurses who balances efficiency with chat and smiles in perfect harmony. As the chemotherapy dose is being started, she and the other nurses always warn the patients to call them immediately if they feel burning in the area where the needle is placed, or if any 'odd' feeling occurs.

I was so used to that speech that I suppose, after a while, I didn't pay much attention to it – a bit like the safety speech on a plane. We all do it: the stewardess begins to talk and we plug in our earphones or start reading the newspaper or simply assume out-of-body mode.

As the Oncology-unit speech is a one-on-one, we all have to make eye contact and pretend to be interested. I did break cover occasionally and say things like, 'Yadda, yadda, okily-dokily, whatever.'

'You must say that in your sleep,' I mused, on that fateful day.

'That and a whole lot more.' Mechelle grinned and shot off to deal with the next patient.

My little space in the Oncology unit resembled a mobile office. That morning, I unloaded my laptop, got out my pen, plugged my phone in to charge and made myself a cup of coffee. Most times I resist the warm fresh scones, croissants and pastries, due to my bowel condensing wheat into cement. That morning, the still-warm, fresh-from-the-oven scones were calling out to me: 'Eat me! Eat me! I won't constipate you for a week! Put lots of butter and jam on me, and I'll be so delicious!' I hadn't stopped at the lobby shop for my usual bar of chocolate, so I gave in and snatched a scone to go with my coffee.

I love bread. Adore it. It makes my eyes roll when I allow myself to eat it. Bread just doesn't like me. Hence the usual denial.

That morning, I'd taken two bites of my scone and a nice sip of my coffee. I felt an odd sensation. Like my hearing was wavering in and out of focus. I got a rush of shivers down my spine. Jesus, I wonder am I coeliac? That scone is making me feel really weird, I thought. Next came a stiffening sensation down my backbone. I would say the hairs on the back of my neck stood up, but I was as bald as a coot, so let's just say I felt a crawling sensation. The sounds in the room began to drawl, the decibels dropping lower than before. Things began to spin. It was like an old-fashioned reel-to-reel tape recorder slowing down gradually.

The next thing I remember, I was waking up and staring at Mechelle who was hunched by my lap. 'What on earth are you doing down there, Mechelle?' I asked, in confusion. As I looked to the left, there was a clear plastic container with 'ANAPHYLACTIC SHOCK BOX' written on it. Mechelle was breathing deeply and administering some sort of injection into my cannula. 'Hang in there for another minute, keep talking.' She was calm and steady, but she was obviously working in a hurry. As the shot of cold liquid made its way into my vein, the sounds in the room returned. The colours changed from blurry and flashy to normal. I became hysterical.

'What on earth are you laughing at? It's not bloody funny! You just went into anaphylactic shock!' Mechelle looked like she was ready to collapse.

'"Anaphylactic shock box",' I managed through giggles. 'All you're missing is the flashing light and a siren on your head.'

'Stop – it's not funny. It can be really dangerous—' Mechelle couldn't finish her sentence. Maybe it was the trauma of it all, but the two of us snorted with laughter. I do remember finding all the colours outside very vivid that day. Whatever was in the antidote shot, I'd recommend it.

The elderly patient in the chair beside me couldn't see what was funny, and sat muttering and blessing himself. Of course, this made me even worse. Knowing I shouldn't laugh makes me uncontrollably hysterical.

Chapter 28

The Score So Far

Cancer 0: Emma 1. I did it! I survived chemotherapy and cancer. I won.

I made it through lots of surgery, I survived chemotherapy. Christmas 2007 was a joyous occasion *chez nous*. Unlike the previous year, Santa didn't bring any game consoles that inebriated adults could possibly injure themselves with, so we could rule out the possibility of my cousin Robyn being impaled on the fireside implements.

A very strange thing happened on Christmas morning, though. Robyn had stayed with us the evening before and we'd had a gorgeous dinner, with more than a tiny drop of wine to accompany our steak. The children eventually went off to bed and we thought it would be a marvellous opportunity to open a bottle of champagne. Then, as there just happened to be two bottles in the fridge, we felt it might be rude not to drink the second.

We all fell into bed, hoping Santa had sorted the presents and was fully organised for the early morning excitement. Needless to say, at six the following morning, when Sacha and Kim bounded into our bedroom to wake us up, that second bottle of champagne didn't seem to have been quite such a brilliant idea.

'Run to the spare room and wake Auntie Robyn. Then we'll all go to the sitting room and see if Santa's visited,' I said, attempting to peel my eyes open and remember who I was and where I had ended up. The last thing I could recall from the previous evening was something to do with a bag of flour.

I shook Cian awake – men have an inbuilt mute button on the entire world when they go to sleep – and we staggered down the stairs, where we met an equally dishevelled Robyn being pulled by Sacha on one hand and Kim on the other.

'Ready?' Sacha yelled, bouncing like a little rubber ball.

'Let's go!' I shouted.

As we opened the sitting-room door, the sight that met us was astonishing. There were white footprints all over the floor and around the fireplace. There were carrots with bites taken out of them scattered randomly around the room and in the Christmas tree.

'Oh, my God, Mum, look!' Sacha exclaimed. 'One of the reindeers pooed on the rug!'

Sure enough, there was a small amount of dung sitting there for all to see. Before you jump to conclusions, a little bird told me that our dogs had actually helped Santa with that idea.

When we counted down to midnight on 31 December, I felt a rush of hope, relief and a massive sense of achievement. I was certain that the new year was going to bring a clean bill of health and a fresh beginning. On that day the previous year, I had begun to feel there was something wrong. I'd had a niggling feeling that all wasn't right where my health was concerned. But I had been so sure that all the sickness must be behind me for good by that stage.

While I'd been having chemotherapy, which is comparable to going on a long-haul flight every three weeks – except that you never actually get anywhere exotic and feel like you've been hit by a bus – to say I got bored is putting it mildly. It wasn't like, what will I do next? I was verging on suicidal. If I hadn't found something new to occupy myself with, I reckon I might be in either the nuthouse or prison. I can totally understand how people become depressed after a long-term illness. For me, the down-in-the-dumps feeling didn't come from questioning my own mortality, pain, sickness or anything physical. My bad times were spawned by sheer tedium.

In the beginning, it was kind of nice to spend a night in a private hospital room, with nobody to annoy me, no dinners to cook, no school uniforms to wash and iron, no arguments over lunch boxes. The fruiters on Jeremy Kyle were kind of interesting, in a morbid-fascination type of way. I could sit and judge and shake my head and tut, while making a smug mental note that I wasn't as dysfunctional as any of them.

At first, the makeover and lifestyle shows were heartwarming and uplifting. To know that a previously body-loathing and introverted person was now able to skip and dance, not to mention wear a wide smile about an enormous photo of themselves dressed in a loincloth plastered on the side of a bus, made me happy. When the days moved to weeks and the weeks turned into months, I changed my mind. I didn't care if Tallulah from Termonfeckin hated her arse. The eight-year-old who'd run away from home to live on a turnip farm with her grandad's boyfriend with the missing teeth and uncontrollable glue-sniffing habit no longer held my attention. I reached a stage where I was so bored with being entertained that my brain was in danger of exploding. I couldn't read another magazine or watch another television programme.

The day can be very long in hospital: rounds start in the middle of the night and breakfast is served soon after 7 a.m. Even the most meticulous shower, followed by body lotion, drying of hair and snail's-pace skin routines were all done and dusted by half past eight. There's only so much walking around the same corridor and past the same ladies on the front desk that can be done, before someone reports you for being weird.

Pressing my nose against the window and counting red cars in the traffic or, if I had a back room, staring at an empty school playground held my sluggish attention for a limited period.

Equally, at home, when everyone else had gone to school and work, my lack of physical ability drove me insane. I would have moments of an energy explosion, where I would haul myself out of bed and insist on trying to clean out the kitchen cupboards. By the time I'd pulled out every jar, tin and packet, I would have to lie on the cold kitchen tiles and wait for some energy to seep back.

'How are you feeling?' Cian would ring to ask.

'I think I'm going to be stuck to the kitchen floor with my own dribble when you get home from work,' I'd whine.

'Why are you lying on the kitchen floor?' Cian tried to keep the irritation out of his voice.

'I was so bloody bored, and I thought it would make me feel better if I wiped all the sticky rings off the bottom of the cupboards,' I explained.

'You should use your energy for something useful. Why, in the name of God, are you even thinking about dirt in the kitchen?'

Of course I had no sensible answer to that question. But I did manage to work out that I needed some low-impact activity to prevent me from going totally gaga.

My mum and most of her family are very artistic. But when I draw a bunny it looks like a turd, people look like spuds and if I deviate from love hearts and symmetrical flowers, which I can create by embellishing a star shape, I'm floored.

In the full of my health, I loved cooking, and particularly baking, but while I was sick I was too nauseous and the cleaning up afterwards was too tiring.

Years ago, when I was pregnant with Sacha, in between all the eating, I started to write a book. Once he was born, the idea was parked. The fact that he never slept for more than a two-hour stretch meant I was mildly delirious with exhaustion for about three years. I was never one of those people who got hammered at parties and swung out of people's sleeves vowing, 'I have a book in me.' It was a little secret. I would daydream about it and wonder how it would feel to walk into the bookshop and see a book with my name on the front. I'm not religious in any shape or form. I would even go so far as to stress that I personally can't comprehend or stomach the whole Catholic ethos that I was steered towards, growing up. But I am a fan of angels – who could dislike something with fluffy wings and a calm serenity? I also want to believe that there is someplace we are all destined to end up. A happy and wonderful place, where there is no suffering and there are endless supplies of chocolate that doesn't give you cellulite. Where there is wine that doesn't give you hangovers and dog's breath the following day. I also believe that most things happen for a reason. I know that what goes around comes around. I'm certain of it. Good things happen to good people. Sometimes it takes a while. Sometimes it's less obvious at first, but I do believe that goodness and kindness prevail in the end. I know that I am lucky enough to have angels or loved ones, or something good and special, guiding me. I have been afforded enough courage, strength and vitality to keep me going during the last few years. And my life has changed for the better, which is not something I thought I would be telling you this time ten years ago.

When I began to write *Designer Genes*, my début novel, it was a sort of spleen-venting exercise. Then it turned into a type of log. I figured it might be useful to Sacha and Kim when they were older, so they could understand what the BRCA1 gene meant and how it had affected me.

I am privileged to have Cathy Kelly, one of the finest authors Ireland has ever produced (of course I'm not biased), as one of the closest people in my world.

Cathy realised I was writing 'stuff' in my laptop. 'What are you writing?'

'Nothing.'

'Show me.'

'No – you're a number-one bestselling author. I can't show you. Besides, it's crap.'

I kept it to myself for a while, and eventually plucked up the courage to show Cathy. She was going away for a family holiday, so at least I knew I wouldn't have to look her in the eye for a few days.

'OK, let's make a pact,' I said. 'If it's embarrassingly dreadful, you can just say nothing. I won't mention it and neither will you. I couldn't bear you having to think of something inoffensive to say. It would be too cringy and, besides, I know you too well and I won't believe you.'

She laughed and promised to be honest.

I still remember Cathy phoning me from the bathroom, where she'd locked herself inside, as the children were jumping on the hotel beds. 'You have to do something with this,' she whispered. 'It needs work and you need to learn about structure, but that's all doable. The story has to be told.'

Cathy was so enthusiastic and encouraging. From day one, she was like my minder. She is now my full-time unpaid 24/7 mentor. With her guidance, I added to what I was writing and turned it into fiction. How she has resisted the urge to mow me down in the school car park, with all the help I've asked of her, I will never know.

To have such a successful author who has many years of experience to hand is an honour and a privilege. Cathy is so giving of her talent and expertise, not only with me but many others. She is patient beyond belief and allows me to pay her in chocolate, coffee and gossip. The first time we met, we clicked. We have been inseparable ever since, and I know an angel sent Cathy to make my life better.

I submitted my manuscript, as they call an unpublished book, and expected to hear nothing for a while, perhaps never. Literally the following Thursday afternoon, I was at home in my kitchen, retching into a pot. Post-chemotherapy nausea, which is like seasickness or morning sickness, doesn't mix terribly well with the smell of meat. Cunningly, I had devised a system where I tied a tea towel around my face to avoid the waft of dinner cooking.

When the phone rang, I forgot to remove the tea towel and answered: 'Hello?' Realising I sounded muffled, I unwrapped my face.

'Can I speak to Emma Hannigan?'

'Speaking.' I scanned my muddled brain. No, I didn't recognise the voice and wasn't expecting any medical results.

'Hi, Emma, I'm calling from Poolbeg. We'd like to publish your book.'

Thank God we can't all be seen on the phone yet. I jumped and punched the air, got a rapid head rush and had to sit down before I collapsed in a heap. I will never forget that moment as long as I live.

I was propelled into a feeling of euphoria. It was a sign that I was going to get through. I just knew that my time was not up. It was proof that, along with the general stuff, like being a mother, I had another important job to do – become a writer. In April 2009 *Designer Genes*, my first novel, hit the shelves, courtesy of Poolbeg Press. Once again, cancer was the loser as far as my mindset was concerned.

My parents bought me a bright pink laptop to celebrate. My little pink 'puter', as Kim pronounced it at the time, became my best friend. I was like that little guy Linus from Snoopy: everywhere I went, Puter went too. I dragged it to the Oncology unit and everywhere else I ended up that year. Book one was finished, so while I waited for the publishing date, about a year after I was first signed up to do the book, I began book two: *Miss Conceived*, my second novel, was born.

My new-found obsession became my solace. When I began to write, the whole world, along with the chemotherapy that often pumped through my veins, disappeared. I no longer fantasised about cleaning the kitchen, sorting out the Christmas tinsel in the attic (in July) or how much dust was under my bed. It was just me and my characters. I believe my writing has saved me. I know I sound like those people who dress in white flowing robes and stand at the edge of the ocean, flapping their arms and bowing to the heavens, but writing has wrapped me in its magic. It is still a dream come true to have a book published. One that goes in real shops, with my own name on the front. I don't think I will ever cease to feel a rush from it. It was a great positive boost for my family too – fantastic to have something more hopeful and cheerful to talk about. The children were so impressed, especially when they heard where it was going to be sold.

'Will they have it in the Bray bookshop, Mum?' Sacha asked, wide-eyed.

'I hope so,' I answered with glee.

Since they were very small, the children have loved going into Dubray Books in Bray. My own mum used to take myself and Timmy to the original shop: it was tiny, with an astonishing amount of stock, and we were allowed to go once a week for a book. Even if Mum and Dad were very low in funds, Mum would beg, borrow or steal to provide us with books.

Timmy was a huge Noddy fan. He would skip in the door and head straight for the Enid Blyton and Ladybird section. The late Mrs Clear, who started the Dubray empire, was in charge of the shop at the time. Each week, she would greet us with warmth. 'Hello, Timmy, how are you today?'

'Hi, Enid, I'm here for your new book,' he would answer. She never told him his real name.

Writing is the one amazing thing that has come out of being ill. I hope I will be able to keep it up for many years to come. It's a true-life example of one door closing and another opening. Who would have thought that getting cancer could have afforded me an entire new career?

Chapter 29

Take Two

Stop the cancer bus, I want to get off.

At the end of January 2008, just as my head began to change from a shiny bald thing to a fuzzy tennis ball, my rash came back. It wasn't as bad as before, but it was definitely there. The pains in my limbs returned too. My fingers felt arthritic and the skin near my fingernails began to redden. My eyelids turned pinky-violet. The warning bell was well and truly sounding. Surely not? No. Not again?

The children had just gone to bed, the fire was lit and Cian and I were sitting on the sofa having a glass of wine. He was stuck into *CSI*, which I can tolerate sometimes, but it's not my thing. Distractedly I touched my face. 'Do my eyelids look red and crusty to you?' I shoved my face into his.

'Is this a trick question?' He looked reluctant to answer.

'No. Either they do or they don't.' I closed my eyes.

'Is this like the does-my-bum-look-big-in-this trick? I'm supposed to say no, or else I get no dinner for a week?' He looked suspicious.

'No. If the rash is back, then the dermatomyositis is back ...' I trailed off.

'Oh. Well, yes, they do look red.'

Searching my body for evidence, fumbling and pressing, like a monkey in the zoo, I got my confirmation. The rubber peas were in my neck again. I also found a clumpy formation under my left arm.

I phoned Blackrock Clinic. 'Hi, Riza, it's Emma Hannigan. I think I've got cancer again. Can I have a scan?'

'You'd better come in and see us, lovey,' Riza answered calmly. Now, I know it's her job to answer the phone in the Oncology day unit, but how that lady is so calm and collected, day in and day out, is beyond me. Nearly every time she answers the phone, it's someone in distress. I couldn't do it. I'd either start crying in sympathy or end up panicking the patient by running up and down and yelling, 'Oh, shit! You're not serious? Fuck, what'll we do?'

A scan was set up for two days later. Within a week, Cian and I were back in Dr Fennelly's office. 'The cancer is back, I'm sorry to say.' Then Dr Fennelly swiftly moved on: 'Your organs are clear once again. It's in the two areas, your neck and underarm, but it's doable. We're not going to panic. Right?'

'Right.' I sat for a moment. 'Do I have to have chemotherapy again?'

'Yes. And surgery. The tumour under your arm needs to come out.'

There were no tears. I didn't try to run around the hospital shouting and yelling. I didn't fling myself on the carpet and thump my fists and feet. What was the point? That wasn't going to cure me.

I guess at that time I could have crumbled. I could have wasted many sleepless nights pondering whether it was fair or reasonable to have cancer again. I could have become bitter and angry, ranted and raved. But I didn't feel the need. More than that, I knew I'd need the energy and concentration to fight again. I had to focus and get through the latest battle I'd been thrown into.

I wasn't as scared as I had been the first time. I knew I could beat cancer. I had proof of that. I had done it once before, so there was no reason why I wouldn't do it again. Taking a deep breath, I spoke: 'Right. Let's go. When can I have the surgery?'

'As soon as possible. I'll organise it for you now,' Dr Fennelly promised.

'How are you doing?' I asked Cian in the car, on the way home from our consultation.

'Well, it could've been better news, but it could've been a hell of a lot worse. At least it's not everywhere and hasn't spread. We'll get through it. You're a pain in the arse, do you know that?'

'Thanks.' I grinned at him. That was it. We were on the rocky road again, but we were still smiling and we were still able to take the piss out of each other. I never worried that we wouldn't make it as a couple. I know it sounds like a dreadfully worn-out cliché, but each hit I took made us stronger. I may have been the one who physically carried the damn disease, but both of us lived through it and battled it – together.

So, I was confident that Cian was on board and just about sane still, but I worried that the whole thing might be too much for the children. I needn't have fretted.

'Henry is back under my arm,' I told them.

'Not him again. I suppose he's Henry the Second.' Sacha raised his eyes to heaven.

'Are the doctors taking him out?' Kim wondered.

'Yes, and then they'll drown him with more chemotherapy medicine.'

'See ya, Henry the Second. Go and get dead with your brother, Henry the First.' They giggled.

I hugged them to me and sighed with relief. I had confirmation that the children had no concept of the implications of cancer. All they did was feed from us. Telling them that I had cancer was the same as saying I had a cold. By the second diagnosis, the words 'cancer', 'chemotherapy', 'oncologist', 'scan', 'blood test', 'neutropenic' were normal to them. Cian and I used the words in front of them. There was no whispering: we didn't have to change the subject when they came into the room. In fact, we made a conscious effort to use the word 'cancer' whenever we could.

'How is your cancer today, dear?'

'It's fine. It's getting taken away by the doctor and put in a jar and poked soon. That's good, isn't it?'

The children would listen and I would see the cogs turning inside their little brains as they gauged our reaction.

I was definitely more upset telling them the second time. I felt I was breaking a promise. I'd said I'd be well again once Santa and Christmas came, and here I was, heading for more tiredness. Luckily little people don't hold grudges. I told them I didn't want to have cancer again, but that it seemed to like me. They accepted that with glee.

'We love you too, so we can understand why it wants to come and live with you. But maybe this time you shouldn't be so nice to it. Then it mightn't want to come back to your body,' Kim suggested.

'That's a good plan. I'll try and do that.' She was pleased to be included in the conversation and, even better, I knew she felt she was helping by making suggestions.

Chapter 30

Hair Today, More Tomorrow?

So, fair enough, now might be the time to assume the utterly-pissed-off-with-life stance. But I haven't come this far to be beaten now.

Definitely because I have an amazing doctor and probably because I'm so bloody annoying, my surgery came around very quickly. I've mentioned before that I have absolutely no patience whatsoever. Of course, I phoned everyone I could until I got admitted.

I ended up going to St Vincent's Private Hospital that time. I met another team of surgeons. Mr Evoy was to remove the tumour under my arm. The breast implant had also shifted on the left side, so Catriona Lawlor was going to replace it at the same time.

As it turned out, the tumour was rather large. Mr Evoy came into my room the evening after the surgery. 'There was a lot of disease there, Emma, I'm not going to lie to you.'

'What does that mean?' I stared at him. 'Did you get it all?'

'Oh, yes. But I was surprised – I removed forty-four nodes.'

'OK. So in the world of nodes, is that a pinch or a pile?' I enquired.

'It's a pile. Sometimes I'd only remove five, ten, maybe twenty.'

'So forty-four is lots?'

'Yup.'

The staff were lovely at St Vincent's, but the elderly building didn't lend itself to luxury or comfort. I won't even start on the glow-in-the-dark crucifix obsession they seemed to have in there. It's bad

170

enough to have to endure post-surgical awfulness, without being subjected to miniature copper men being tortured.

I'm glad I knew about my morphine allergy or I reckon I would have had 'Always Look on the Bright Side of Life' singing in my head as the little metal man sprang to life in a drug-induced rendition of the Monty Python classic. Mercifully, the hospital has been rebuilt and is a totally different place today.

Once I'd recovered from the surgery, I was straight back on the chemotherapy bus. Just prior to starting my new poison, a small discussion broke out. Pathology at St Vincent's were sure the cancer they had tested was breast cancer. But, to put a spanner in the works, Blackrock Clinic's pathology lab thought it looked more like ovarian cancer. I found this fascinating.

Dr Fennelly reminded me that a patient cannot be given the same mix of chemotherapy twice. So, in other words, every time you get a six or eight months' cycle of chemotherapy, it has to be a different mix of poisons.

'That's mad, Ted,' I said to Dr Fennelly – I was being Dougal from *Father Ted*.

Second time around, the stuff I was to have would kill breast and ovarian cancer. So it was win–win all around – for me, not the cancer: Henry the Second would be well and truly dead.

The second mix of medication didn't cause alopecia. In fact, most new forms of chemotherapy don't make your hair fall out. The fuzz on my tennis ball continued to grow, and before long it even began to look like hair. Alarmingly, it was dark and seemed to be trying to get all curly. 'But I'm a blondie with poker-straight hair,' I said to the oncology nurse.

'Very often, hair grows back looking different. At least it's growing back – and evenly at that.'

'Oh, don't get me wrong, I'm thrilled. Even if it was leopard print, I'd be delighted. It's just odd. I'd say my follicles got such a shock at being fried and frazzled last time, they're all curling in terror.'

Chapter 31

Chemotherapy – the Sequel

Please, God, tell me it's going to work this time. I feel like the living dead – this is so toxic it must be working …

The second bout of chemotherapy was a bastard. No other word for it. Perhaps I was actively trying to make good my promise to the kids not to welcome the cancer, but I was gonzoed. I was exhausted and lost a lot of weight. I was utterly disgusted the first time: all that medication and all I lost was two miserable pounds. Like most women, I spend a lot of the time denying myself the stuff I'd like to eat. We all know it's wrong to eat doughnuts for breakfast, but it doesn't stop them tasting good.

The first time I'd had chemotherapy, a friend had come into the Oncology unit to keep me company. Dr Fennelly came around to have his usual meet-and-greet with me. I introduced them, and Dr Fennelly asked me how I was tolerating the medication. 'Have you been managing to eat?' He rubbed his chin. I think he was being kind in even asking me this question. At that stage I was so bloated and puffy, I looked like I'd been pumped up with one of those automatic pumps they use for bouncy castles.

'Yes, I'm still eating away. Why?' I asked.

'Well, one of the side effects of this particular one is a loss of appetite.'

'Oh, can I have some, then?' my friend piped up.

'Not enough to make her hair fall out – she has to go to a wedding next week. Just enough to make her want to eat half a rice

172

cake a day for a while. She's bought a very pale pink dress and she'd love to lose a few pounds so she doesn't feel like a raw white pudding in it. What do you say?' We both looked at him expectantly.

He laughed, but mentally he must have been booking a double room for my friend and me at the funny farm.

By the second go, however, I changed my mind: I'd lost too much weight. I looked scrawny and, God forbid, ill. Nothing I usually liked tasted good. I had to force myself to eat. I knew that if I didn't have a good, balanced diet, I would never get better, but it was hard.

'I should be ecstatic, I should be revelling in the fact that I can sit and have lard dipped in chocolate for breakfast, but I don't want it. I look like a sick person,' I moaned to Cian one evening.

'You are sick. You have cancer again, you goon.' He smiled.

'You do know I'll be that ancient person in the nursing home in many years to come who complains about all the "old" people, when I'm eighty-five.' I laughed.

But that was the whole point. Even though I was fighting cancer for the second time, I didn't see myself as ill. Fair enough, I would go to the Oncology unit, have chemotherapy, do my injections at home to boost my immune system and take anti-nausea medication, but I wasn't really sick. Not in my own head at least.

'Just so long as you keep thinking along those lines, you'll be fine,' Cian managed. We were sitting at the kitchen table sharing a cup of coffee.

My older brother Timmy walked in. 'She won't be going anywhere, have no fear. Believe me, I tried to get rid of her for years, and it didn't work.'

As I've said before, family and friends are the key factors when you're fighting an illness. I am blessed to have both nearby any time I need them. There are so many people I can call and I know they'll be there for me.

There is one thing I cannot stress enough. Talking. Whether you're ill or not, sharing your thoughts with other people never fails to help. If you're going through cancer and you don't feel comfortable talking to those closest to you, try a cancer support centre.

If you're having a really dreadful day, when you feel you can't cope and nothing is making you smile, rent a funny movie. I know that sounds like the most feeble advice, but you can't beat sitting back and relaxing, with a bit of laughter thrown in. Besides, everyone knows it's rude not to eat sweets, chocolate and popcorn while you're watching a movie. Even though I wouldn't touch one now if you paid me, I found Jelly Babies delicious while I was having chemotherapy. Oddly enough, numerous other oncology patients agree with me. However it works with the change in taste – perhaps some crazy chemical reaction – I reckon Bertie Bassett has some indirect influence in chemotherapy production. I always have friends on the Oncology ward when I have a party-sized bag with me. I know money can't buy you love, but when you're having chemotherapy, handing out Jelly Babies guarantees a smile.

Chapter 32

Friday the Thirteenth

Friday, 13 June 2008: a horror movie – starring me. If this day is supposed to be an unlucky day, it's living up to its name. Have I travelled back in time? Are we in the Dark Ages? Help!

I would talk for Ireland. I believe I even talk in my sleep. But this has stood to me. I don't carry things around feeling burdened or isolated. I get it out there, and for me, that works. I have also run into what one might class as 'difficulty' because of my outspoken nature. Myself, Cian, the children and my parents went away for a weekend down the country. We thought it would be a break from the constant routine of trotting in and out of the hospital.

I felt we'd hit a wall. Like gerbils on a wheel, we'd been enduring my sickness, surgery and treatment for so long, it might be a welcome relief to hire a house and go away for a couple of nights. We found a self-catering cottage with enough space for us all, packed the car and set off. We'd been hoping to have a little adventure and a bit of diversion.

Big mistake. If I ever have chemotherapy again, which I hope I won't, I will stay within a ten-mile radius of Blackrock Clinic until it's finished. When we arrived at the cottage, we unloaded the car and went out to a local place for a meal. I didn't enjoy the food and had to force myself to eat. I didn't even want dessert. By the time we got back to the house and settled ourselves in bed, it was quite late. The following morning I woke up feeling like my heart was thumping through my chest. I was so hot and febrile I could barely move. I could hear Cian's and the children's voices in the kitchen.

'I brought you some coffee.' Dad appeared by my side.

'I'm sick, Dad. We have to call the nearest hospital,' I managed to croak.

Dad flew into action, phoning Blackrock Clinic. My temperature was at 38.8°C, so it was too dangerous to risk driving back to Dublin. Well, that was what we believed at the time. In hindsight, it would have been less risky to run naked up one side of Kilimanjaro and travel backwards strapped to a skateboard down the other side than what I actually had to do.

Cian and Mum planned a little trip to distract the children, as Dad and I sped, with the guidance of Mrs Satnav, to the nearest public hospital. The foyer was huge, bright, airy and modern. A bit like the open-space part of a new shopping centre. I was lulled into a false sense of security.

'Wow, this place is impressive, isn't it?'

'Let's hope they have the medical expertise to back up the space-age lobby.' Dad strode ahead, full of mission.

I was to discover that the entrance was actually the best part of the entire place. The A & E department was so disorganised and noisy with frenzied staff and irritated and panicked patients, it made for a shockingly rude awakening.

'Hello, I'm here with my daughter Emma Hannigan. We phoned ahead to say we were coming. She's got a neutropenic infection and is shivering badly,' Dad explained.

'We don't do queue-skipping because you phoned. If we did that, sure the place would be in chaos,' the gum-chewing, bored-to-tears woman at the desk answered.

'If this isn't chaos, I'd hate to see what they consider messy. What else would it take to move towards chaos? A suicide bomber?' I whispered to Dad. I felt nervous and isolated. I realised I wasn't able to cope with the whole illness thing when I wasn't surrounded by familiarity. Getting to know your team of caregivers is vital. Once you have established that you're having treatment in a particular place, you should make a huge effort to get to know the staff. Bribe them with boxes of chocolates and packets of biscuits, if necessary, but make yourself known and get to know the doctors and nurses in return. At least that way you can feel a sense of security and confidence.

All my illusions of hospitals were shattered when I entered Hell on Earth. Up until that point, I had no idea that some specialists still have the God complex. This is when they stride along corridors with Queen's 'We Are the Champions' playing in their heads, while the imaginary wind machine blows their hair. They are ten feet tall, and the rest of us are scabby vermin, scuttling around, hoping to be stood on. I shit you not, these people, most of whom are men, still exist.

'Does your head hurt?'

'Pardon?' I couldn't understand his line of questioning. We were in A & E and I had explained that I was having chemotherapy treatment and I had a temperature of 38.8°C. Once the thermometer shows anything over 38.0°C, it's showtime according to Phil, my blue friend on the chart. You must rush yourself into the nearest hospital, as it indicates an infection. With my usual neutrophil level of zero, I knew that the shakes and fever could spell serious danger.

The protocol at any other hospital I'd experienced had always been:

1.   Isolation (as in, a private room).
2.   Immediate vital signs checked, i.e. temperature, blood test, blood pressure.
3.   Immediate verbal assessment, which involves asking the patient questions and then, funnily enough, listening to the answers.
4.   Immediate intravenous antibiotics to cover the obvious infection.

More often than not, I would also receive a saline drip to make sure I wasn't dehydrated. I had stupidly thought that this procedure would be common practice in all hospitals when a chemotherapy patient presented.

This smug git seemed to think I needed a totally different approach. Either that or he had always wanted to be a neurosurgeon and had missed the exam or had been told he was to work for ten years in A & E for some dreadful misdemeanour in a past life.

'Do you have a headache?' He didn't look at me, he just kept shouting.

'I have a throbbing head, but I think that's due to the fever rather than anything else,' I answered.

'Wait here,' he barked. I wish I'd had the energy to yell at him that I was hardly in any fit state to go anywhere else.

I sat in A & E for two hours, shaking and hoping I wouldn't die of infection or have my bag stolen. The hospital was like the land of the living dead, containing what seemed to be the most bedraggled and inebriated members of society concentrated in one space. Luckily I was so hot and sick – my eyes were rolling in my head – that I managed to fit in with the other patients. Eventually, a foreign man came and stood by me like a sack of wet sand. 'Emma Hann-gin-anne?'

'Yes,' I wheezed.

'Come, you do scan.'

'What do you mean a scan?' I was totally confused.

'I know nothing. Man just tell me to bring Emma Hann-gin-anne. You are him?'

'Yes.'

'OK, good. Walk now.' I looked at Dad in a slightly panic-stricken manner.

'I suppose you'd better go. I'll wait here,' he vowed.

'If I'm not back in two hours, you can assume I've been dismembered with a chainsaw and put in small jars for clinical research.' I sighed.

Before I knew it, I was having a brain scan. Now, maybe the man thought I was totally mental and needed confirmation that I should be locked up for life. Or else he was the seventh son of a seventh son, born at sea with a caul on his head, and had the ability to see inside bodies with his bare eyes. Perhaps he had noticed, via his X-ray vision, that I had a tumour the size of a large grapefruit on the frontal lobe of my brain, and knowing he had to back up his revelation by some sort of medical procedure, he was doing a scan to prove his point.

'Did the consultant see some massive tumour while he was staring at me earlier?' I asked the radiologist.

'I don't know, love. I'm not paid to have an opinion, I just operate the machine. Lie down, please.' The radiologist left the room.

What felt like a year later, I was wheeled back to A & E. Dad was pacing up and down, looking like he wanted to murder someone.

'Here's your dinner.' A female with a grey, furry face (very sweet on a three-week-old kitten, not so cute on a grown woman), bitten fingernails and a bad, bad attitude banged a rubber tray in front of me.

'I think you're mixing me up with someone else. I didn't order food.' I forced a smile as I seriously began to wonder if I was suffering from acute memory loss, coupled with a crippling dose of split personality. Why were all these things happening to me that I knew nothing about? I hadn't asked for a brain scan and I was certain I hadn't ordered any food.

'Well, I'm giving it to you. There's nothing more being served in here until seven tomorrow morning.' Before I could attempt to get to the bottom of the oddness, Furry Face had gone. It was four o'clock in the afternoon.

Dad raised the pink rubber dome that covered the plate of food on the brown rubber tray. There, looking embarrassed and terrified, was a curled-at-the-edges sandwich, filled with startling pink stuff perching on a slick of spreadable margarine.

'Is this a joke?' I stared at Dad.

'Well, I'm not laughing.' He rubbed his face as he exhaled loudly. I placed the rubber dome back over the sandwich, so I didn't have to look at it any longer.

By ten o'clock that night, I was still in a ward, separated from my vomiting neighbour by a torn curtain. Two car-crash victims and a man suffering a vicious asthma attack occupied the other beds.

I was too bloody ill to care, but Dad was becoming more and more distressed. I haven't exaggerated the scene – if anything, I've dulled it down.

By the time I was wheeled to a private room, which smelt strongly of fresh vomit, I was exhausted. 'I need to take my medication,' I told the admitting nurse.

'Oh, no. It's ten o'clock,' she said.

'What's that got to do with anything?' I was getting really pissed off with the nasty attitude every member of staff seemed to have in this hospital.

'We give drugs out at six and after breakfast in the morning. That's it.' She began to walk away.

'But I take medication four times a day.' I was aghast.

'Not here you don't, unless you want to use your own.' She stood with her hands on her hips and stared at me with impatient disdain.

So, incredibly, that's what I did. I self-medicated the entire time I was in that public hospital. I could have been taking heroin ten times a day, and nobody bothered to check. I had a large zip-up bag of medication, and not one person ever looked inside it. They didn't establish exactly what was causing my high temperature and were blindly treating me with a broad-spectrum antibiotic – which is standard procedure – yet they never cross-referenced with the medication I was giving myself. I know quite a bit about my own medication, in so far as I can readily count out dosages and know what time to take stuff, but I'm not a doctor. I have no training or specific information on which drugs go with others.

I spent two nights in the isolation room. Get this: it had an enormous flat-screen television on the wall, yet there was no bulb in the bedside light, and the blankets had holes in them. The paint was peeling off the walls and it was dirty. Would it not have been safer to have a clean, functional room with no expensive television?

My children were not allowed to come and see me. My friends were told to stay away. Cian and my parents were permitted to enter the room, one by one, if dressed in disposable gowns, masks and gloves. Of course we all understood the reason behind this: I had a severe infection, which could essentially kill me. We had no quibble with that. But the whole thing became utterly ludicrous when the food came around. The catering lady burst in the door with the trolley, dumped my food down, left the door open and trundled off. She wasn't wearing so much as an apron, never mind gloves or a mask.

Do you remember the SARS virus that swept the world in 2002 and 2003? It kicked off in Guangdong, a province in China. Within three months, it had infected thirty-seven countries, with a case fatality rate of 9.6 per cent. Even though serious measures were put in place by the World Health Organisation, they couldn't figure out how the disease was spreading so quickly. An observant passenger put two and two together as he sat on a long-haul flight. The air stewards were passing food, drink and duty-free goods from passenger to passenger.

The reason I'm telling you all that useless information is that I could easily have come a cropper due to the lack of a consistent isolation policy in that public hospital. It made shag-all difference that the doctors, nurses and my family were dressed like survivors from a nuclear attack. The entire effort was futile when one person who was in contact with every illness in the place wasn't following suit.

Even though I was very ill, on a drip and oxygen and feeling as bad as it's possible to feel, that lady did serve one purpose: she made me laugh like a banshee.

When the oncologist eventually came to see me, two days after I'd been admitted, we didn't hit it off too well.

'May I ask why you ordered a brain scan the other day?' I wondered.

'I was doing routine checks. Not that you need to know why I do my job.' He glowered at me nastily.

'Excuse me?' I looked at him in disbelief.

'You do not need to question my actions. I am the specialist.' He looked more than a little affronted.

'I am a patient, not an amoeba. I will not stand for being spoken to like that. You are the most unpleasant and unprofessional creature I have ever had the misfortune to encounter. Your staff are mean and your abhorrence for your job spreads through this place quicker than the cancer you attempt to treat,' I said.

This unnerved him and made him do a Basil Fawlty jump backwards, but it was only the beginning. He went a dreadful shade of puce and stuttered about Dublin people and rudeness. 'You have no respect,' he roared.

Ha! I thought. Talk about pot and kettle!

'In order to gain respect, you must earn it.' I eyeballed him. Before I was ill, I was outspoken, but I would never have argued like that.

181

After many years of being prodded and poked, I guess my bullshit-o-meter was at an all-time high.

Unfortunately for both of us, I was incarcerated on his Oncology ward until my antibiotics kicked in. I hated that man on sight – not Christian of me, but that was the truth of the matter.

I had the intelligence to refrain from starting a really big row with him. I was paranoid he might try to put arsenic in my drip or hold a pillow over my face at three o'clock in the morning. I assume it was mainly due to my outburst that I was moved by an uncommunicative nurse into a large ward later that very day.

All the other patients there were gravely ill. There was a constant gargle from breathing-apparatus and other life-support machines. In the bed next to me, there was a tiny old lady. She was lying very still and hadn't moved for far too long. Just as I was deciding she was no longer with us, she began to vomit.

I pressed my call button repeatedly. Nobody came. I pressed it again. Nothing. Eventually I shuffled into the hallway. At this time, I was dizzy and febrile, not to mention oozing with hate for the hospital and the God-complex git of an oncologist. I made my way down the corridor to a small desk area.

'Yes.' No eye contact, no smile. Two nurses sat at the nurses' station doing paperwork. Neither even looked up at me. I firmly believe that attitudes in any business come from the top. If the boss is a prick, the employees will also be arseholes. This was most definitely the case in that hospital.

'The lady beside me is vomiting and she's in a bad way. I pressed my call bell but you didn't come.' I assumed they would jump to attention, full of apologies.

Neither batted an eyelid.

'As you can see, we're busy. We'll come when we're good and ready.' Now I had eye contact. In fact I had a what-are-you-going-to-do-about-that-then smirk.

Unfortunately, what followed can only be politely described as an explosion in my brain. Boom! I yelled like a woman possessed in that hallway. I shouted a string of curses that would have impressed my son's friends no end. I spat out words I didn't even know were in my vocabulary.

The result was that the nurses sauntered towards the old lady and simply mopped the sick off her clothes. Astounded, I watched them leave her in that state. They didn't try to soothe her. They barely spoke to her and quite clearly didn't give a toss about her.

'Where are your clean clothes?' I began to root in her small brown Formica locker.

'I don't have any,' the little sparrow managed to answer. Mine were all T-shirt material nightshirts with supposedly cool slogans like 'I got an A in shopping' on the front. Her own stained one was an old-fashioned flannel style, with flowers and buttons to the neck.

'I know you'd probably rather not, but will you use one of mine? It's clean at least. What anti-nausea medication are you taking?' I asked. 'I'll get the nurses to bring it.'

'I'm not taking anything. They give me a bag of stuff when I get the chemotherapy, but I'm always sick like this a few days after treatment. That's why I have to stay in for a while.' She vomited again, and was left dry retching and bathed in sweat against her soiled pillows.

I learned she had no family close by, due to the closure of so many cancer services in Ireland. It's probably illegal but, with her permission, I looked at the chart that was clipped to the end of her bed. Sure enough, she was not taking any anti-sickness tablets. As I had a large bag of mine in my locker, I took some out and showed her. 'I promise I wouldn't give you anything that would harm you. You're on the same type of chemotherapy I did last year, and I know these won't interfere. Please take one. If it doesn't help, that's fine. But if they work, you can have them.'

At first she regarded me with suspicion. But she was so nauseated and weak she decided to trust me. With a papery, shaky little hand, she took the tablet and swallowed it. Together we hobbled to the communal bathroom and removed the soiled nightwear and changed her into my Minnie Mouse one. For the first time, she smiled. 'I feel like a young one!' Her twinkly eyes glinted as she looked down at herself.

'You'll be doing the can-can up the hallway in a minute once that tablet works its magic. If you get your leg up high enough, you could kick one of the nurses in the face,' I suggested.

We rolled out of the bathroom giggling like schoolgirls.

Later that day, when I asked the consultant why the elderly lady was not on anti-nausea medication, he told me to mind my own business.

'It became my business when she was left in such an inhumane state earlier on. I'm not asking for her personal banking details, I'm simply enquiring as to why in this day and age any person should have to endure such sickness when anti-nausea medication is readily available,' I hissed, refusing to be bullied by him. He told me she was a public patient and those tablets were too expensive.

Later I chatted to the lady again, and urged her to seek an alternative hospital. We discussed the options and figured that there was another public hospital only a little further from her home town. 'It would be worth the extra few miles to try another place,' I said.

She agreed. 'I think I just needed someone else to point it out to me,' she admitted. Sometimes, even if the care is dreadful, it can be really hard to have the courage to move. But there is always a choice. If you are not being given the care you feel you need and deserve, try another hospital. If I hadn't asked for a second opinion in 2007, I might not be alive today.

Go with your gut instinct. If you're ill and you feel you're not being listened to, move somewhere else. I know the choice has been limited with the closure of many centres of excellence around the country, but we all have the right to a second opinion. It may take a bit of travelling and initial hassle, but it could save your life.

Whether you are in the public or private system it makes no difference. You always have the right as a patient to request another physician. There is never just one person in the entire system available to you. Hospitals and doctors may not always encourage patients to make waves and ask for another opinion, but that doesn't mean you can't insist on one.

Never let any illness silence you. Speak out and you will be heard. You mightn't make a lifelong friend in the doctor you leave behind, but the oncologist I encountered in that hospital isn't someone I'll ever invite for dinner. Neither will his name ever be found on my Christmas-card list. People who don't show human empathy and professionalism shouldn't be tolerated. You only have one life: don't allow bullies to ruin it. I have attended many hospitals over the last few years and the unpleasantness I met in that one was unusual. It is not acceptable to be made to feel sub-human. Being ill is bad enough without being treated badly. Exercise your rights as a patient, and find a hospital where you will be better cared for. Again, in L'Oréal's words, you're worth it.

I didn't spend a moment longer than I had to in that establishment. I was able to walk away and I obviously lived to tell the tale. But I can honestly say that those few days were up there with events like funerals in the enjoyment stakes.

Chapter 33

Laughter Is the Best Medicine

Along with perhaps Xanax, vintage Bollinger and a week in the south of Spain.

Most people who have survived a crisis in life will agree that having a sense of humour during darker times is vital. Back in 2007, during a particularly low point in my treatment, my children made me laugh like a drain – in public. Their gleeful innocence worked as a thera-peutic alkali on what would have been a horribly acidic period without them.

Some people are conscientious objectors to the circus. I understand that it's cruel to make wild animals perform. Neither should they be kept in cages and made to travel. But the one I took my children to in 2007 was lovely.

The performers were beautiful, raven-haired, Italian-looking people. The tent was not much more than a Wendy house with an extension. The wildlife hadn't been captured on the African plains. There was a dozy, overfed rabbit and a badly behaved pony with a very long fringe and a tendency to bite the ringmaster. Neither animal was made to talk or wear a glittery G-string. In fact, the only way the humans could stop the pony grazing in the middle of the ring was to bribe it with a bag of apples.

The entire audience consisted of Mum, myself, the two children and five other people. The running of the show was fascinating. The sparkly lady who served as ticket seller was also the shopkeeper and an acrobat. The ringmaster multitasked as the magician, the ice cream seller and the other half of the acrobatics team. The other two members of the cast were clowns: one was tall and thin, like a string of spaghetti, the other like a stocky macaroni curl, with the height of a seven-year-old.

'Why is there a child doing the clown job?' asked Kim. She was six at the time.

'He's not a child, he's just small.' I hoped she'd be quiet.

'But he's the same size as me.' She was intrigued and totally baffled.

'He's a little person,' I explained. I could literally hear the cogs turning in Kim's brain. That wouldn't be the end of the conversation, of that I was certain.

The show passed off fairly peacefully. Between flashing, spinning yokes, popcorn, ice cream with that alarmingly neon lime-green colour dashed through it and the admission cost, we'd spent the guts of that month's mortgage money. But we all tried to bear in mind that these people were keeping up a dying art. They were making a huge effort to entertain all nine of us, with never-faltering smiles, God bless them.

On the way home, I had to stop off at the supermarket. As I wrestled with the welded-together line of trolleys, a growling, rust-riddled old banger clanged to a halt beside us. The back window was rolled down and out tumbled the horizontally challenged clown. I felt Kim stiffen beside me. Then she bolted towards the man and cornered him.

'Are you a Munchkin?'

Now it was my turn to stiffen.

'No, lady.' He smiled graciously. 'I am what you say meejit.' He grinned as his Italian accent tried to get around the word.

'What do you eat?' Kim asked gravely.

'Pasta, bread, eggs, usual stuff,' he nodded, not a bit put out by the very direct questioning.

'Don't you need small things like a cat does?' Kim wasn't about to let this interview opportunity pass her by.

'No, I'm exactly like a normal person, just smaller.'

I had to interject: 'Everybody's different, but that's good, isn't it?' I couldn't stand by and allow her to continue talking to him like he was from outer space.

I could hear the cogs in both of my children's brains starting to turn.

Sacha, who'd been silent to that point, came forward. 'Do you wear nappies, or can you go to the toilet like a real person?'

'OK, you don't need to answer that.' I felt sweat beading my brow and panic setting in. This would end in offence if we didn't move away – and fast.

'Don't worry, Mr Idjit.' Kim patted his head as if he were a gerbil. 'Our mum is a bit different too. Look – she's bald.'

Before I could stop her, Kim pulled off my wig, complete with small, pretty skullcap, revealing my boiled egg of a head.

Luckily the clown was a step ahead of me. He rapidly made his escape.

I cried laughing the whole way around the supermarket that day. It still makes me giggle.

I am blessed – or cursed – with a dark sense of humour. This is something that has stood to me over the last few years. As my hair began to sprout again, during the second year of chemotherapy in 2008, my wig became a bit slippy. And itchy. The soft fuzz of hair acted like a skating rink for the meshy material inside of the wig. This in turn caused the wig to twist around and very often the fringe part would end up at my ear. This rotation happened especially when I was weighed down with shopping bags, with two children galloping towards reversing cars in the supermarket car park. My son Sacha, being a sensitive sort, would often appear at my side and yank the wig back into place. We thought this was normal in our house. Passers-by, though, would freeze at the sight of a child moving his mother's hair around.

The flip side of having cancer, the treatment and side effects, is humour. Hand on heart, I can safely say that cancer has afforded me some of the best laughs imaginable. There is a wonderful light that creeps forth, like a beacon, just when you feel you can't take any more negatives.

My wig, for instance, had a life of its own. I'm certain it has eyes and snuffles around in the dark at night when we're all asleep. It has been worn by everything from teddies to our poor long-suffering cat. One incident that will remain with me until the day I die took place on the Stillorgan dual carriageway. It's one of those roads that never sleeps. It has four lanes of heaving traffic, pretty much 24/7.

I was on my way to Hotel Blackrock, sitting at red traffic lights. It was quite cold outside, and I am the type of person who likes to make my car into a sauna. I had the seat heater on high – probably warm enough to slow-cook a casserole on a long journey – and the automatic blow heater was at 26 degrees. The children were going through an obsessed-with-Michael Jackson phase, so I was jigging away to 'Billie Jean', head bopping and fingers tapping the steering wheel, when I got a fit of the itches. This was like having lice (not that we've ever had those in our house), mixed with a bag of feathers, dancing on your skull. The wig feels like it had been doused in itching powder or has tiny electrodes attached to it, creating thousands of little pinging and darting prickly sensations.

My usual ploy, especially in public and daylight, was to make my hand into a claw and dig my fingernails into my irritated scalp at intermittent stages. If the tickling was very bad, I often had to resort to the other method: both palms held flat on my head, moving the wig back and forth very slightly and slowly. It had a soft-sandpaper scraping effect. Doing this is quite acceptable in your own company, or with someone who knows you really well.

On that occasion, the itching was so violent, I instinctively shoved both hands into the sides of the wig at my ears. I lifted it off my head. It flipped over my forehead, down my nose and into my lap. I scratched like a lunatic. Oh, the relief was wondrous. The lights turned green and I put my foot to the floor. I'd had no chance to scoop my wig off my lap and yank it back onto my head. When I glanced into my rear-view mirror, the driver of the car in the adjoining lane was rooted to the spot. The shock on that poor git's face still makes me laugh.

My wig now lives happily in a drawer in my dressing room. Don't feel too bad for it, though. It still comes out for special occasions and has done the rounds at drunken dinner parties. It has also featured in many a Facebook profile photo. It's been taken on dates to quite a few fancy-dress functions and has helped several male friends to pose as drag queens. It's no longer needed on a daily basis, but it will always have a special place in our family.

While I was having chemotherapy, and indeed radiation, my immune system used to plummet, as I've mentioned, and I was saddled with UTIs, or urinary-tract infections. It's like having a sieve for a bladder and a bag of stabbing feathers living in your nether regions. I've taken so many antibiotics, but UTIs still seem to weasel their way into my body. The most soothing thing to drink is cranberry juice. It actually works. Asparagus is also incredibly effective for soothing the infection.

On one memorable occasion I woke up in the middle of the night, wondering why everyone in my dream needed to go to the toilet. As I peeled both eyes open, I realised that my bladder was going to explode.

'What's wrong?' Cian muttered, on autopilot. He has this astonishing ability to chat, then instantly resume corpse-type sleeping. I, on the other hand, wake up for five seconds in response to a noise and am awake for the rest of the night, only falling asleep fifteen minutes before the alarm clock is due to go off.

'I'm bursting to go to the loo.' Stumbling to the en suite bathroom, I stubbed my toe and walked into the door jamb. To say that I peed like a donkey is putting it mildly. I got back into bed thinking I'd have the best sleep ever. Wrong. The pain in my back started. It was like being kicked by the donkey who'd had the pee. Then the dreadful tingling feeling took off – that I-really-need-to-pee sensation, but when you get there nothing happens.

I was wide awake with no hope of sleep at 2.30 a.m. I tiptoed down the stairs to start drinking pints of cranberry juice. Just in case you were wondering, it's much less painful to pass large amounts of urine rather than a dribble. By morning, I'd drunk two litres of the stuff. In between trotting in and out of the bathroom, I was uncomfortable and spiking a temperature.

It usually takes me twenty minutes to get to Blackrock Clinic from my house, especially if I leave early in the morning. Knowing the journey wouldn't take too long, I went to the bathroom, then flew into the kitchen and drank a last glass of juice.

Bad mistake. Every annoying person in the world was on the road that day. Learner drivers and tiny old people with bottle-end glasses, who could barely see over the steering wheel. They were all out in force. Every single light turned red as my car approached. Every inch of road that could possibly be dug up had a group of high-vis-vested men with protruding arse cracks.

By the time I was halfway there, I was jigging uncomfortably. After forty minutes in the car, I was strongly considering abandoning it and dropping my trousers in the middle of the motorway. Well, it did have a grassy bit.

I have seat heaters, as I mentioned before, which might have encouraged me to just 'go' and the heater would dry the mess, but the paranoid part of my brain worried that I might be electrocuted, the seat would blow up and I'd be found dead, with a fried bum and soaked in my own urine.

By the time Blackrock Clinic came into view I was nearly crying. All the jigging, bouncing and trying to think of other things were not enough. I became so frantic that I started opening all the compartments between the two front seats. My car was a Volvo at the time, and the person who owned it before me put everything from television screens to a fridge inside it, literally.

I clicked the fridge open. It was wide and deep enough for me to sit on and just go – but I could see a motorised wheel whizzing around to show the thing was working. I would have had to perch up there in full view of the entire lane of traffic. I actually wouldn't have cared about angry businessmen seeing me squatting over my fridge – but, again, I didn't want to fry myself to death. After all the surgery and cancer treatment, it would have been remiss of me to kill myself with my own piddle. If I was going to top myself, I owed it to my family and my doctors to do it in a much more dramatic and glamorous manner.

Instead, I saw a break in the traffic, so I zoomed down the bus lane. This is one of those roads that the police hide on regularly. They seem to gain immense pleasure from booking people going to hospital. Bizarre. That morning, even if they'd followed me with ten squad cars and a whole team of motorbike guards, they wouldn't have caught me.

At the hospital entrance, the barrier that doles out the ticket was working like a rusty cog. 'Come on, come on,' I yelled into the dispensing box.

I pulled up and parked diagonally in two spaces, yanked the keys out of the ignition, grabbed my handbag and ran as fast as my legs would carry me.

'Coming through – red alert,' I yelled, as I flung my coat and bag at the reception desk.

The nearest bathroom was the disabled one just behind the main reception. I scuttled in, managed to disrobe just in time and hoist myself onto the seat, which just happened to be about five feet off the floor. As I was flopping onto the toilet, eyes watering wildly with the pain of peeing and a feeling of tremendous relief, one of the receptionists kindly spoke through the keyhole.

'I'm closing the door for you, Emma. I'll call a doctor now – you're obviously very sick. Don't worry, pet, we'll sort you out. I have your bag and coat safely with me.'

It was a few minutes before I had the courage to get off the pot. Not because I was embarrassed: I was just terrified that if I tried to walk the two flights to the Oncology day unit, I'd need to pee again.

I walked like John Wayne to the reception desk. 'Oh, girls, I have the worst waterworks infection of my life. I think my bladder's trying to come out my belly button.' I slumped on the desk like a wet rag. 'I was so close to wetting myself there that I was going to have to let it go and ring you to come and give me a surgery gown at the car.'

'Surgery gown? Ah, no, we would've given you some scrubs. Matching trousers and top. It's too cold to go around in a surgery gown.' They giggled.

I still haven't totally discounted the idea of keeping incontinence pants in my glove box for future such emergencies.

I spent that entire day in the Oncology unit banging on the door to dethrone other patients. There is only one toilet, which is unfortunate when you have a bladder like a leaking sieve. I got more antibiotics, and it sorted itself out. The girls on the reception desk and I laughed like hyenas, which prompted a frank discussion about how awful it is for women when we have to pee. Men can pretty much go anywhere. They can even go in a bottle if they have to. Aim out the car window or into their manbag, if they carry one. But women are at a distinct disadvantage with the whole thing. I do remember reading about a plastic device like a wonky funnel that would enable women to pee into jars or similar vessels at festivals, but I don't think it ever took off. At least none of my friends have ever admitted to owning one. But, the good news was that by the end of that day, just like a good episode of *Sesame Street* in the seventies, I did learn a valuable lesson: it's not a good plan to cross a urinary-tract infection with a pint of cranberry juice and early morning traffic in a big city!

Chapter 34

All in Vein

Percy the port, please! Cancel that notion of becoming a successful junkie. My veins have had enough.

As I reached the halfway stage of chemotherapy phase two in 2008, my veins held up a white flag. Once an axillary node clearance is performed, this means that some or all of the lymph nodes in the underarm area are removed and the arm on that side can no longer have pressure applied to it. This essentially means that blood pressure can't be checked, blood samples can't be taken and chemotherapy can't be administered. The other arm must be used, or the leg can come into play for blood-pressure cuffs.

My right arm looked like it had survived a week's holiday with Edward Cullen and his vampire family. Between the chemotherapy going in and the blood coming out, I was like a three-week-old banana.

'I would recommend having a port put in,' one of the nurses advised.

I was brought to the little examination room off the Oncology day unit, where I met 'the torso'. He is that old joke – what do you call a man with no arms, no legs and no head in a swimming pool? Bob. This was rubber Bob. Medical-demonstration Bob, to be exact.

Bob also had a scary removable chest wall: it was a flap of pliable, skin-coloured rubber, which could be lifted to reveal his innards and his port. The port was basically a round metal contraption, about twice the size of a one-euro coin, with a line ending in a needle.

The needle went into the jugular vein at the base of Bob's neck. He had no head, as I mentioned, so in reality, the needle went into his stump.

'Will I have to go around with that plastic line hanging out of my chest for the whole time?' I eyed the thing sideways with horror.

'No, not at all. The port is invisible on most patients. At worst, all that can be seen is a circular shape. The line just looks like a little vein going along your neck.'

Of course, the port had to be put under my skin, which meant a little operation. A small incision would be made, the port would be positioned, I would be stitched back up, and Bob's your uncle. Or your new port, in my case. Each week, instead of stabbing my poor violated arm, the nurses could put a needle and a line into the port instead.

I went home to talk to Cian and the children about it.

'What's the port's name?' Kim asked. As usual, everything and everyone had to have a name.

'What about Paul?' I suggested.

'No, he's our uncle.' She looked at me as if I was mental.

'Percy,' Sacha stated.

Percy was scheduled for insertion the following week. I was to go to the Cardiac unit, as the surgeons down there were equipped for Percy insertions.

'You'll be sedated, not totally knocked out, and you won't remember a thing. Just the same as if you were having a scope,' the surgical team explained.

I lay on the blue gel mat on the surgical bench in theatre. It's like a huge, flat cooler-bag insert. The drip was inserted, amid plenty of rubbing and slapping of my hand in an attempt to raise the poor bruised veins.

'They're hiding because they know the drill now. If they show themselves, you'll stab them. Not as thick as they look, my veins,' I joked.

Even healthy veins hate the cold. That's why your hands look all lumpy and veiny when you're hot and sweaty on a sun holiday. The heat makes them rise and protrude. Equally, if your hands are freezing cold, they go numb and the veins sink.

I got my sedative and the surgeon came in to start the job.

'Good morning.' He was expecting me to slur like a wino.

'Good morning,' I answered.

'You seem very awake.' He seemed a little surprised.

'That's because I am very awake,' I answered.

We discovered that it takes rather a lot of juice to send me to the Land of Nod. On this occasion, I had decided that, so long as I couldn't feel the pain, I would prefer to stay awake. The more anaesthetic I had, the more hungover I would be afterwards.

It's not a hangover I relish – like the type you get after a night of over-indulgence, when you've been out for dinner or dancing like a mad thing on some shiny dance floor. With an anaesthetic hangover, there's a horrible sluggish feeling without any of the fun from the night before.

Local anaesthetic was injected, which feels stingy at first, just like at the dentist. After that, there was just a sensation. The noise of cutting flesh was vile, but the job was done in a matter of minutes. I was sewn up, and Percy was ready to rock and roll.

I was sore afterwards, especially when the port was accessed the following week for blood samples and chemotherapy. This involved a nurse opening a whole bag of tricks – a blue disposable picnic pack of fun. Lisa, one of the oncology nurses, gave me one for Kim to play with, which she adored. Inside she got little vials of saline solution, a plastic kidney dish (why are they kidney shaped? Why not heart- or Mickey-Mouse shaped?), plastic tweezers, cotton wool, plasters, disposable gloves and a big pink bottle of antiseptic stuff. It was all a fantastic bundle of play fun.

The area around Percy – my skin – was wiped with the pink alcohol-smelling stuff, using the tweezers, cotton wool and disposable gloves. I was itching to have a play too. But apparently I needed to qualify as a nurse to be allowed do that. Then a vacuum-packed needle with a long plastic line and a bit of Lego was pushed into the centre of Percy. There's a short, sharp jab as it pierces the skin, but that's it. Pain over.

The port was a saving grace for a long time. My arm was allowed to heal. The worn and bruised veins were able to recover. I could rest assured that the chemotherapy and bloods could be done with ease. Before, it could take the girls three stabs to access a vein properly.

My only problem with Percy was the insurmountable 'ick' factor. He never did anything to me. He never insulted me, pooed in my airing cupboard or called me Fat-arse. But I hated him. Because I was very slim back then, Percy was visible in all his glory under my skin. I looked like I had a grey metal bottle cap poking out from the top of my collarbone. The line that was pretty much invisible on other patients protruded quite noticeably.

'Why have you got a straw coming out of Percy?' Sacha asked.

'That's so he can give a drink of chemotherapy to Mr Jugular Vein. Then Mr Jugular Vein feeds the chemotherapy all around my body, so it can look for Henrys and kill them,' I explained.

'Cool.'

It was pretty cool, especially when I was so low and sick. But as my chemotherapy came to an end, Percy became my pet hate. None of my clothes covered him. It got to a stage where I was buying things to wear, not because I loved them or they suited me, but because they covered up my port. I vowed that I would have Percy removed just as soon as was humanly possible.

Chapter 35

Almost There

I can virtually see the light at the end of the tunnel – it's glinting and winking at me. Wait! I'm coming. Last stop on the way – just a few minutes in the dying hole.

It was the middle of October 2008. I pitched up at Blackrock Clinic for my second last treatment. As I waited in the hallway to have my blood taken, I had the pleasure of meeting a wonderful young woman. She was the same age as I was – thirty-six.

She was there for a routine check-up, including a blood test, along with her tiny bundle of joy.

'Congratulations.' I smiled instantly at the little sleeping bunny in the high-tech buggy.

'I still look at him and have to pinch myself.' Her eyes shone.

'I know – it's amazing being a mum, isn't it?' I joined in with the misty-eyed wonder of it all.

'Well, I was told I might end up infertile due to my chemotherapy, so he's an extra miracle.' She'd been single and childless when she was first diagnosed.

'How did you cope on your own?' I was fascinated and full of awe.

'Well, I was never on my own. My friends and family were great,' she continued, 'but I did fret and wonder would I have any chance of meeting someone. I felt I would be damaged goods. Who would want a bald, barren bird, when they had the choice of plenty of healthy versions with hair?'

I was quick to point out that she hadn't been even grazed with the ugly stick. That girl was stunning: dark skin, glossy hair, long eyelashes. There was not a hint of sickness or that she'd been through any kind of trauma.

'The fact I met my husband when I was bald and coming out the other side of treatment still astounds me,' she confided.

'Why? Because you felt so low about yourself?' I probed.

'Yes, and because I wasn't even that sure of how to socialise once my treatment was over.'

This was an issue that had never even occurred to me. I have been fortunate to have been protected by the cocoon of Cian, Sacha and Kim. I had the whole husband-and-kids package sewn up before I had to begin my battle. But so many people have to do what I did, and then get themselves back out into the big bad dating world. I had another one of my major moments of clarity as I tried to put myself into the situation this girl had been faced with.

Imagine going into a pub with a friend and meeting a nice guy. He chats to you and everything seems to be going well. He asks for your number. Me being me, I would be so tempted to blurt out my life story in a sentence – right there and then. 'You can have my number, but you need to know this is a wig. Look, I'm really bald. My breasts aren't real and I've just finished chemotherapy. Did you want to have children in the next two weeks – because I'm infertile?' Can't imagine I would have found a husband too quickly, can you? Most single people who finish treatment must feel a degree of that. What is the right thing to do? Wait until you've had two dates before you're comfortable enough to scratch your head and dump your wig in your handbag?

I asked this new mum all those questions.

'At first,' she bit her lip, 'I wasn't sure how to handle it. I did blurt out my cancer story in a tirade just once, but then I learned the best policy was to lie.' She shrugged her shoulders and smiled. 'Basically, I only went out in a group, for short bursts of time, in the beginning. I made sure there were at least two close pals with me, who knew the truth.'

'And that gave you more confidence?'

'Of course, and at least I could go into the toilets and scratch my head and have a quick chat with a close confidante, then go back out to the pub or club or wherever we were and continue being a young, free and single "normal" girl.'

'Wow,' was all I could utter.

Until her energy and hair returned, she just took it in baby steps. When people asked her what she did for a living, she lied about that too.

'Well, saying I wasn't working at the moment because I'd just finished chemotherapy was a bit of a conversation-stopper. So I used the recession to my advantage. I said I was between jobs.'

'Good call, and nobody batted an eyelid,' I nodded. She had met her husband nine months after she finished treatment. He was accepting of her possible difficulty with conception, and they never looked back. He was the right person for her.

From mulling this predicament over, and without meaning to sound like a smug married person, I think that's the key. Cian has stood by me through thick and thin, through fat and thin, and through thin, bald and eventually fuzzy-headed. But I believe he is the right person for me. I am just blessed that I found him many years ago. If I had been married to the wrong person, I can't imagine our marriage would have survived the journey.

I waved goodbye to the smiling new mother with her precious cargo and thanked my lucky stars yet again that I had my hubby and children. To add to the euphoric, positive air, I was excited about the fact that I was so nearly there. My chemotherapy was two doses away from being over. I decided to celebrate by going to the coffee shop in the next-door building. Their coffee is so strong, I'm sure you could dance a mouse on its surface, and it gives a good pep in your step.

I found myself in the lift with an elderly couple. I noticed I'd walked out of the Oncology unit with my pen in my hand.

'Do you know where the CT scanning department is, dear?' the elderly lady asked.

'Sure. We're heading in the right direction. I'll show you the way,' I volunteered.

As we came towards the right department, I explained where they needed to check in and sit.

'What time will my wife be finished at? I need to tell our son to come back,' the old man asked.

'You'll have to ask the lady at the check-in desk. She should be able to give you an idea.' I smiled and gave them a little wave as I proceeded to walk towards the coffee shop.

'Typical doctor! Just because I'm not your patient, you won't help me.' The man was quite cross and indignant.

'Oh, no, you're mistaken. I'm not a doctor.' I must have looked very surprised. 'I'm a patient too – I'm just going to grab a coffee.' I gestured towards the café.

'But you're carrying a pen.' He looked me up and down in confusion.

I suppose I've spent so much time in Blackrock Clinic over the years that I've developed the familiarity with it that the staff have. If they would like to offer me a job and pay me handsomely, I will gladly march around with my pen five days a week! Imagine if I acquired a white coat and a clipboard as well. I could be the greatest unqualified specialist in my field.

As I was due to finish my chemotherapy less than six weeks later, I thought it would be safe for Cian and me to go away just for one night, without the children.

'Hi, I've decided we should go on a little night away. Will you book somewhere?' I asked Cian on the phone. (I told you before, I have no patience!)

'Eh, riiiight. Do you think that's a good plan? Should we not wait until you're over the chemotherapy? Remember the last time, when you nearly stabbed the horrible oncologist in the hospital where they torture elderly ladies?' he reminded me.

'Ah, yeah, but that's all in the past. We're almost at the other end of this, so it'll be fine,' I assured him. Famous last words.

What happened? You guessed it. We ended up doing a lunchtime dash to a country hospital. I affectionately called this one the Dying Holes. Have you seen *Madagascar*? It's an animated kids' movie about wild animals raised in captivity in New York City Zoo, which will make you laugh out loud. One of the characters – voiced by David Schwimmer – a.k.a. Ross in *Friends* – is a hypochondriac giraffe. He believes that he is dying all the time and has convinced himself that he needs to dig a hole and sit in it, waiting to die. Hence him dubbing it his 'dying hole'.

I visited the human version of the dying hole during that particular infection. I waited in the hallway to see the oncologist on duty. The basement area was lined with plastic chairs, manufactured purely to make people's arses numb within seconds, while simultaneously chilling them from head to toe. The large plastic slots at the back of each chair served two purposes, as far as I could make out: they caused a huge draught and made sure the seats were astonishingly sore to sit on. Those chairs were about as comfortable as a marble slab. Perhaps they were trying to prepare our bodies for the morgue.

There was no piped music, television or other distraction. Not even a badly tuned radio station with a twelve-year-old DJ broadcasting dreadful underground rave music from his own garden shed.

I sat down alone, as my husband was parking the car. Nobody looked up or even sideways.

'Terrible, isn't it?' an elderly lady muttered to nobody specific.

'Yes,' another victim answered.

I sat in stunned silence, trying to retract my head into my neck in the hope that I might become part of the wall and thus invisible. Please, nobody look at me. I don't want to get into a bless-us-and-save-us-isn't-the-world-awful conversation with depressed pensioners I don't know.

Just to put you in the picture, it was November and it was sleeting outside. It was brass-monkey temperature, with a wind-chill factor of minus a toe, if you stood in it for too long. Yet each and every one of those people was totally bald.

I tried not to do open-mouthed staring in rigid astonishment. Did their particular forms of cancer also kill the temperature receptors in their heads?

There seemed to be a uniform of pale grey T-shirt material tracksuits, all to be worn four sizes too big. I find pale grey a dodgy enough colour to pull off at the best of times. In my humble opinion, only people who are dark and under the age of twenty can look good in said garments. But when you have that dreadfully unbecoming yellowish-green hue that only a chemo patient can muster up, they're not flattering. I'm not saying all of this to be bitchy or personal. Oh no, it's because this, to me, represented giving up.

The entire two hours I sat there was like having my toenails removed with pliers, minus any anaesthetic. Not one of the people had a single positive thing to say. There was no smiling, most definitely no laughing, and a total sense that the cancer had won. The air was defeatist and negative. I had to zip my lip and sit on my hands to prevent myself exploding like Captain Caveman. I wanted to shout and yell at them all, 'Why don't you hang up bunting and wave white flags, and throw a party for the bloody cancer altogether? Give it presents and pat it on the back?' I have read so many articles about cancer and the importance of attitude, how positivity can boost a patient's outcome by up to 30 per cent.

That is significant. I will probably be condemned by many for even writing the above sentences. I know the charitable way of looking at those poor sick people is to embrace their actions. They have enough going on without having to wear a wig or dress in their finery. 'Leave them alone – don't be so shallow,' I hear you cry.

But I can't stress enough how different I always felt when I pushed myself to make an effort. Some days, due to my autoimmune disease, it took me up to two hours to have a shower and dress myself. By the time I'd managed to put on make-up, I'd have to lie down again to recover. But it was worth it. I could pass a mirror at home and not feel like jumping off the nearest tall building. In case I sound utterly vain, that's not what it's about – I'll never be a candidate for Miss World. This is about self-esteem and confidence, which are vital. I don't think that all sick people should go around skipping and delighted to be ill. That's crazy. Neither do I think that all patients should drop the fight. Put on your jeans and a nice shirt. Wear the dress that makes you feel special. These are things that cancer shouldn't be allowed to steal from anyone. All I can say is this: by painting on my smile – literally – my eyebrows and a 'healthy' complexion, I felt more normal. I didn't feel like a victim. For me, as a living young woman, that was crucially important.

You don't need to sit in the dying hole. There is no rule that forbids you to feel OK about yourself. There is no rule that says you have to let the cancer invade your psyche as well as your body.

Cancer does not have to destroy your hope. It can kill some good cells, it can make you feel like you're dragging your arse around the place like a dead slug. It can make you crave a burst of energy. It can even make you forget how it feels to be well. That's all normal. That's par for the course. I get that. But don't let it quash what's inside. Nothing can take away your hope and inner spirit. Not unless you allow it to.

That day in the Dying Holes hospital, I only needed an antibiotic and I could leave. I had severe pain in my ear, so the doctor was satisfied that was the cause of my temperature and I was allowed to go. I ran out of the place, jumping and waving my arms around. 'What are you doing, oddball?' Cian tried to step away from me and pretend he didn't know me.

'I'm living!' I shouted, like a woman possessed. 'I am not dead. I am living,' I yelled at two men who scurried past me.

Cian and I fell into the car, cackling.

'We'd better drive really fast before you get locked up.' He grinned.

I sped away from the Dying Holes, invigorated. Fair enough, I'd added another course of drugs to my already rattling system, but they would kill the infection. I would feel fine again in a few days. It would pass. It always did. It was transient – but my inner vigour wasn't. To this day, I don't allow cancer to quell my spirit. No matter where this illness takes me, and no matter how many times it tries to attack me, it will never dent my inner core. When cancer decided to mess with me, it picked the wrong girl.

Chapter 36

Round Two to Me!

Updated score: Cancer 0: Emma 2. And now can we all live happily ever after?

Eventually, in December 2008, the chemotherapy ended for the second time. Dr Fennelly wanted me to stay on a maintenance dose of a new drug called Avastin.

'What's Avastin when it's at home?' I asked.

'When cancer forms, the reason it manages to spread so rapidly is, first, due to the speed at which the new cancer cells grow. Then, second, it creates its own independent blood supply, which has nothing to do with the body's regular system,' Dr Fennelly explained.

'So it's Cancer Central. Its own little rail network that can fly around your body in no time?' I mused.

'Precisely. Avastin is like a seeker drug. It goes in through the vein and searches for this particular little evil blood supply and cuts it off.'

'Dead. Finito. Brilliant or what? I am constantly bowled over by all the amazing stuff that scientists and doctors discover with regard to cancer, but this sounds like the best one yet. God, imagine being clever enough to think of inventing that stuff,' I marvelled.

'All tumours are either hormone-positive or hormone-negative. For the hormone-positive ones, we can use Herceptin. But your tumours are all negative, so that wasn't an option for you. Avastin could work really well for you, Emma,' he said.

I was thrilled. I was to go every three weeks to the Oncology day unit, have a blood test and, assuming all was well, they would give me a bag of Avastin magic juice.

You might wonder why I was delighted at the prospect of more drugs through my poor sad veins and the promise of indefinite blood tests on a three-weekly basis. Quite apart from the constant medical intervention, I would have peace of mind. I would have another little minder, helping to stave off the bastard cancer.

Score so far: Cancer 0: Emma 2.

Oh, yes. We like it! Now that the cancer had been drop-kicked again, I had to move on to another thing. I became obsessed with having Percy evicted.

In September 2009, I got an early birthday present. Percy came out! I was wide awake again and able to have a running commentary from the surgeon. 'Here it is!' He held it up for me to see. I gave Percy the fingers, but I didn't offend anyone, as my hands were covered by the theatre gown.

Now I had a scar where Percy used to lie. I have so many slashes and gashes on my body that it's beyond a joke, but I reckoned I'd go and have this one softened by Dr Condon and his magic Fraxel machine. Bye-bye, Percy, hope we never meet again.

Meanwhile, my non-cancer life took off in a totally different direction once the chemotherapy had stopped. I did radio interviews in conjunction with the publication of *Designer Genes*.

Ireland's TV3 gave me my first ever taste of television. I was lucky enough to be asked on to *Ireland AM*, the early-morning show, with Sinéad Desmond and Mark Cagney. I spent the entire night before the show doing twinkly-eyed staring into the darkness. But this was a new kind of wide awake in the middle of the night: this was excitement, nerves and sheer terror – but in the best possible way. Everything from the make-up and hair to the lights and cameras enthralled me. Here was I, an ordinary young(ish) one from Bray, on the television!

The biggest turn of events happened on my birthday, in September 2009. I was in the queue in Starbucks, waiting for my chai tea latte, which doesn't smell or taste like normal tea – if you haven't ever had one, you're missing out – when my mobile phone rang. It was the researcher for *The Late Late Show*! I said, 'Oh, my God,' so many times that the old lady in front of me turned to ask me if I was all right.

'It's the people from *The Late Late Show*, they want me to go on.' I gestured madly at my phone.

'Are you going to do it?' She looked me up and down, her tiny prune face poking out of her tightly tied headscarf. Her expression was deadpan and totally devoid of expression.

'What do you think?' I asked, biting my lip – of course, it's perfectly normal to ask a random stranger with a tartan shopping trolley if one should accept an invitation to appear on *The Late Late Show*.

'Ah, do, you might as well. They've never rung me.' She collected her coffee and dragged her shopping trolley off to a table.

As fate would have it, I had bought a bright-pink evening dress only an hour beforehand. The lady in the shop had asked me where I was going in it. 'Nowhere that I know of – I just love it. I love the glittery straps at the back. I think I have a bit of a shopping illness,' I had confided. As she'd wrapped the evening gown in delicious pink tissue paper, I'd had a brief moment when I considered seeking professional help with my shopping habit. Luckily Cian doesn't examine my wardrobe on a regular basis, quizzing me about new arrivals. In fact, he has so little interest in clothing, I don't think he'd notice if I went out dressed from head to foot in gold lamé with feather adornments.

'Don't we all?' She sighed, resigning herself to the fact that some women need to shop.

So that just proves it: shopping for no apparent reason at all pays off. Imagine if I'd had to go on *The Late Late Show* with nothing to wear. The shame of it. So, ladies, being a shopaholic is a good thing! I will never forget my thirty-seventh birthday, being on the most famous and iconic chat show in Ireland with Ryan Tubridy. It was an utterly mind-blowing honour. Most definitely an experience that I'll cherish forever.

So, you see, having cancer was beginning to turn my life around. I used to hear cancer survivors say that being critically ill changed their lives for the better. That puzzled me. I wondered why they hadn't gone and organised a bungee jump or flung themselves out of a small plane or hiked up a sheer mountain face. Apparently that sort of stuff gives shedloads of satisfaction and improves people's lives no end. Could they not have improved themselves without getting sick? I can understand the whole process now. It's not the actual sickness that causes the transformation. It's the aftermath. It's the eye-opening, striking realisation that life is for living. That each day is precious. That we only get one bite of the cherry. That we should live for the day.

I know I sound like a stick-waver now. 'Feck off and stand on top of your own nearest mountain in flowing white robes, flapping your arms around and yelling at the seagulls,' I hear you cry.

Believe me, I am, in many ways, one of the most cynical people you will ever meet. As you know, I don't do the religious thing and I don't believe in alternative medicine or rubbing yak droppings on my skin to make me well. But I have copped on to the fact that life is short. I've had that wave of gratitude that I'm still alive. Maybe I should be at mass twice a day. Maybe I should never eat cooked food, meat or shellfish when there isn't an 'r' in the month. Maybe I should be scaling tall buildings in a bikini in New York in December and pushing myself to the limits.

Maybe then I will have a rock-solid guarantee that I'll never get cancer again. But that's just not me.

So life had returned to normal, which I adored. I was back being Mum with energy. I was able to get through a day without feeling I needed to have a quick snooze on the gravel on the way from the car to the front door. I no longer had to go to bed by nine in the evening, feeling as if I'd spent half an hour being beaten to a pulp by a frenzied cage fighter. I remembered what it was like to feel normal.

I was managing to swim, cook dinner, do the grocery shop, wash and iron the clothes, write books, publicise them and even go out for dinner or drinks when the occasion arose. I was well again. I had done it. I'd beaten cancer twice. Cue the bluebirds and the Disney music.

Chapter 37

Ding-Ding: Round Three

The first two instalments were such a hit, my body's decided to make a sequel to the sequel.

In 2009, for the first time ever, I realised I needed to make sure that I factored some me-time into my life. I'd gone through the wonderful yet bloody exhausting mission of having two babies very close in age, followed by a ridiculous amount of service in various hospitals. By now, Sacha and Kim were nine and eight respectively, and for the first time in so long I found myself exhaling. It was as if the mist was clearing, and I was finally able to see a clearer path ahead.

We all know exercise is good for body and mind. I know that in my own case especially, taking all the drugs into account, it was vital that I kept up swimming. Truthfully, I would rather do a three-hours solid session of ironing rather than exercise, and I loathe ironing. After the mastectomy, I was very stiff. I had been warned to take it easy while stretching.

'You will have to be very careful doing certain things – for example, hanging clothes on the line,' I was told.

When I had the axillary node clearance two years later, I was warned about lymphoedema. 'Lynda who?' I felt confused. Yet another long, cumbersome name to get to know. It was slotted into the words-that-sound-like-they-were-invented-just-so-people-can't-pronounce-them-or-know-what-they-mean part of the hard drive in my brain.

'This is where lymph, which is fluid, can get trapped in the arm.

Once a lot of lymph glands have been removed, the fluid builds up and causes swelling. This swelling makes the arm stiff and sore and in turn can make it hard to use successfully,' the medical people in the know told me.

In English, it's like the hosepipe that carries this lymphatic fluid has been cut. So the hosepipe (your arm) can get blocked. This makes your hand and forearm look like uncooked dough and feel kind of stiff. It's not pleasant – when it happened to me, my hand looked as if it would be nice to squeeze or stick my finger into, to see if it made a dent. But it hurt like hell and felt really tight.

So, my once-normal arm looked like an elephant's trunk after it had been shamelessly bashed with a lump hammer. Not the most attractive thing to behold. My lymphoedema wasn't bad – it wasn't at a stage where I would have made money at the circus – Mr Idjit was safe. But it set off alarm bells. I knew I wasn't supposed to have a raw French stick for an arm.

In line with my newly aware thoughts of finding some me-time, I figured I should sort out the puffy-arm syndrome. I found a wonderful lady called Deborah Fernandes who performs a treatment called manual lymphatic drainage or MLD. This is like a very gentle massage, which essentially moves the lymphatic fluid and keeps it flowing freely. Deborah is a chartered physiotherapist and has many years' training in oncology treatment. She studied this specific type of MLD under a man called Professor Leduc. I would recommend MLD to anyone who has had a mastectomy. But I would make sure the person is a chartered physiotherapist and obviously check with your oncologist first. (That paragraph is like the fast-spoken bit at the end of a radio ad, where they tell you, 'Terms and conditions apply'.)

The second thing I had to do regularly, which, as you know, I don't enjoy, is exercise. I know some folk love it. I married my polar opposite when it comes to exercise. As I mentioned before, Cian is Sportacus. He does triathlons, half-Ironman and Ironman races, and has even managed to convince himself he enjoys them. Himself and his friends actually think it's normal to go cycling for five hours. He enjoys running in the snow and swimming in the sea, and would go stir-crazy if he couldn't train every day. My mother is cut from the same exercise-bunny cloth. If she's not on a horse, she's walking dogs, doing Pilates, gardening or in a pool for aqua aerobics.

I, on the other hand, would happily use a mobility cart to take me to my car so I could drive to the postbox and back. Hand on heart, I would never have an overwhelming urge to pull on a Puffa coat and go for a bracing walk. However, due to my early menopause, I need exercise to maintain bone density. Due to all the drugs I've taken, I need to be aerobically fit, so my heart doesn't stop and my liver doesn't become hard and refuse to work. Due to the amount of chocolate I consume, I need to exercise so I don't resemble a raw white pudding with eyes.

In October 2009, I arrived at Deborah's place for a massage. As she moved her fingers around my neck, she stopped. 'What's this?' She looked grim.

I put my finger on the spot she was concerned about and my heart stopped.

'Shit,' I stated. The rubber peas were back.

I left Deborah, promising to keep her informed. I phoned Dr Fennelly that evening. I have always maintained that any medical query should be dealt with immediately. I never wait and hope it will go away. I don't mull it over and decide to put it on the long finger. All things have a better chance of being fixed if dealt with NOW.

Dr Fennelly saw me the following morning. Only three weeks previously, I had been momentarily thrilled to receive clear CT scans. Had I managed to reach November, I would have had a full year without cancer – for the first time in three years. 'We'll remove them, but you'll have a small scar on your neck,' he told Cian and me.

There was a brief silence, before Cian and I burst out laughing.

'Sorry, I shouldn't laugh, but she's hardly going to mind a small scar at this stage.' Cian nodded towards me.

I've had so many bits removed that I call myself the human patchwork quilt. Instead of feeling lowered by, or even ashamed of, my scars, I have a sort of bowing respect for them. OK, fair enough, it would be more aesthetically pleasing not to have any, but my zips represent my survival.

On 30 October 2009, Mr Magee came to my service once again.

He removed the infected lymph nodes (Henry the Third) and, once again, parts of my body went off in a jar to be inspected by Pathology.

I waited ten days for the results. The waiting time is what I hate most. I brought my mobile phone to the toilet with me. I carried it to bed at night. It was worse than waiting for a boy to ring when I was a teenager.

I kidded myself on and off during those ten days.

'Surely I can't have cancer again,' I said to Cian. I had somehow figured that twice was enough for anyone. But deep down, I knew. The warning signs were also there. The rash was spiking on my eyelids again. My arms and legs were sluggish when I swam. The dermatomyositis was struggling to raise its ugly head. Hand in hand with Mr Cancer, his girlfriend Ms Dermatomyositis was looking to party. My neck was their ballroom.

The morning Dr David Fennelly phoned me to tell me the pathology lab had tested the nodes brought welcome relief. To see his name pop up on the screen of my mobile phone ended the torture. 'Emma, there's cancer in those nodes again.'

Even though the news was not what I'd wished for, at least I knew. For me personally, not knowing and having to speculate was vicious. When I'm left teetering on the edge of a proverbial cliff, I can't cope. Being kept in the dark is the most destructive thing for me.

I am so fortunate that my doctors, Dr David Fennelly, Dr Frances Stafford, Dr Michael Moriarty, Dr John Armstrong and many others, have been marvellous at keeping me informed. I have no doubt that they would love to see me well, even if solely to get rid of me. I ask questions all the time. I phone constantly when I'm worried. I write down my questions so I don't forget what I need to know. If I'm in a panic, I just arrive at the hospital and find someone to talk to me: a medical professional who can answer my questions and put my mind at ease. I don't allow fear to silence me. I push it away by talking to people who are in a position to give me the answers I need.

These clever and learned medical people have saved my life. Pure and simple. Every time I have been sick, they have jumped to support me with their amazing medical minds and their unstinting human support. I know I am blessed to have these brilliant people minding me.

When I got the confirmed cancer diagnosis for the third time, my first thought was that I didn't really have time to do the cancer thing again. I was working on the edit of my second book, rereading my third book and putting the finishing touches to the fourth.

'We're going to do some radiation therapy this time,' Dr Fennelly informed me.

'Fantastic! Research!' I responded. 'I've had chemotherapy twice so I need a bit of radiation to balance it all out.'

'As the nodes we're dealing with are isolated and close to the surface of the body, radiation will sort them out. The previous times you've been diagnosed, there were too many areas to cover. This time radiation will be a good option,' Dr Fennelly explained.

Let the fight recommence, I vowed inside. This certainly wasn't what I had hoped for. I had honestly thought that twice might be enough for me with the whole cancer lark, but obviously my battle wasn't over just yet. So be it. I hadn't come that far to be knocked down. I was more determined than ever to win.

If cancer wanted a fight – let it just try. I was standing at the crossroads with my arms open wide. Bring it on.

Chapter 38

A Pink-Ribbon Day

My own personal pink-ribbon day! Have you ever had one of those uncontrollable urges to do something insane?

I sat like a mannequin in my car. I'd just hung up from my conversation with Dr Fennelly. 'Bugger it anyway,' I said out loud to the steering wheel.

My thoughts drifted to my family and friends. I would have to tell everyone the cancer was back. I hated upsetting people. Just like the two previous times, that was the part I loathed more than anything. I had such wonderful support and genuine love from so many people, I detested having to deliver more bad news.

I told my family individually and did the quickest thing I could think of for everyone I knew. I sent a text message again. I know that might sound like a dreadfully cold and abrupt thing to do, but picture the scene. I've already done the coffee mornings, the endless phone calls, the reassuring of me and other people, and the positive clichés not once, but twice. There's only so many nods and ah-wells we can do. To make it easier for everyone, I sent a text explaining that, although the cancer had tried again, it was now safely in a Kilner jar and I was having three weeks of radiation. That was that.

The final line of the text read:

I feel positive about my outcome and I would like you all to be the same. Onwards and upwards. Emma

All my friends responded accordingly, with best wishes and lots of kisses. But the predominant answer was, and I quote, 'Holy fuck'. I thought it was eloquent and, in that particular instance, fitting.

I went for my swim because I was having a virtuous day. As I paced up and down the pool, I had a sudden overwhelming compulsion to do something mad. I contemplated going to buy a Chanel handbag or Jimmy Choo shoes. But, as usual, I'd spent more than I'd earned that month. A little ping noise went off in my head. I would get a tattoo. I nearly drowned as I flailed towards the steps. I dashed into the shower and ran out of the place, hair still wet.

In Bray, they have an award-winning tattoo shop – or is it called a parlour? It is alleged that Britney Spears had a tattoo done there. And Cian had once come home with the back of his entire calf engraved with a swirly Maori tribal drawing. So I knew Atattooed was the place to go.

Now, you might think I ought to have had enough of needles, what with the chemotherapy, all the surgery and the endless blood tests. But I like to think of myself as open-minded. All needles shouldn't be tarred with the same brush. The other way of looking at it, and the psychoanalysts among us could tell me it carried a whole other meaning, was as my way of controlling a needle for a change. Yadda, yadda. Quite honestly, it was like a bolt from the blue and seemed like an utterly marvellous idea at the time.

'Hello. I would like a pink ribbon on my wrist, please.' I shrugged my shoulders with excitement.

'OK. I'll show you some designs and you can choose one, or we can draw one for you,' the girl explained.

We discussed size, shape, shading and position. All very specific and informative. All sorted. It wasn't going to cost a fortune either, so we'd be able to pay the mortgage and feed the kids. It would last forever, so it was fantastic value. Much better than a designer handbag, of course.

'We're booked up until the week after next …' The girl was still smiling and flicking through the pages of a very heavily marked appointment diary.

'What?' I was bereft of smiles and probably physically jumped backwards from the counter. 'But I want it now.' I knew I sounded like Veruca Salt from *Charlie and the Chocolate Factory*.

'Oh dear. Sorry, but our guys are very well known and it takes a while to get an appointment.'

As I was about to throw myself on the floor so I could heave and sob and work myself into a full-blown tantrum, the phone rang. It was someone cancelling a job at two o'clock that very day.

'Can I come in then?' I was standing far too close to the girl's face – I'd say my eyes were like those of a small furry animal after a sugar injection.

'Erm, I suppose so.'

Before she could change her mind, I paid in full and skipped out the door. After my compulsory bar of chocolate and some wickedly strong black coffee in a nearby café, I sat smiling in a squinty-eyed, knowing way at the other customers.

Two o'clock came around very quickly. Feeling small-person-on-Christmas-morning excited, I returned to Atattooed.

'Have you a reason for getting this?' Badger asked. Yes, that was his name and, no, he didn't look like one.

'Yes, I'm celebrating getting cancer for the third time.' I smiled.

Confusion flashed fleetingly across his features.

'Oh, no, it's OK. It's been carved out and I'm having a few goes of the radiation machine and I'll be back on track. It's third time lucky for me.'

Badger seemed to get my reason for wanting my little pink ribbon. Now it sits proudly on my right wrist and has little twinkly conversations in a high-pitched fairy voice with the pink elephant on my ankle. God bless it, the pink elephant was the only tattoo on my body for a long time, so it probably needed a bit of counselling to accept its new sibling. I'm hoping they'll grow to love each other.

When my husband came home that night, instead of us having to sit and have hushed conversations about what a pisser it was that I'd somehow managed to get cancer again, we admired my tattoo. I diligently rubbed nappy cream on it for a week, as instructed, and I'm delighted to inform you that it's still very happy there.

Chapter 39

Project Radiation

*... with two new tattoos thrown in for free. What more could a
girl ask for?*

It was November 2009. The radiation therapy began the week after
my pink ribbon arrived. I was told I would need three weeks of
treatment. At first I wasn't sure if that meant I needed to stay in
hospital for three solid weeks. I had no concept of what radiation
was or even how it was conducted. Would it be in a gas chamber
or on some sort of torture rack?

To my huge relief, it was an in-and-out job, which only takes a
couple of minutes each time. The biggest hassle was dragging myself
in and out of St Vincent's Hospital in Dublin every day. Before the
'fractions', as they call the sessions, (in my case fifteen fractions would
make up a whole treatment) could begin, I had a quick CT scan.
This was to determine the exact spot that would be zapped.

'Oh, I like your little pink bow.' The radiologist grinned. 'At least
you're OK with tattoos – you won't be too alarmed by ours.'

I smiled, but inwardly I was slightly puzzled. What on earth was
she mentioning tattooing me for?

I was bloody stunned when she jabbed me with a needle, making
two tiny black marks, one on the side of my breast and the other
in the middle of my breastbone. Now, it wasn't about the marks,
because at that stage, unless it was a large hoof-shaped brand in the
middle of my forehead, I couldn't have given a toss. With my scars,
two tattoos and God knew what else, my body wasn't going to be

chosen to model on the catwalk in Paris – but I was still rather shocked. I had never heard anyone mention a permanent tattoo in conjunction with radiation therapy. Maybe I'd been hiding under a rock or perhaps it's that so few people chat about cancer treatment openly, but the tattoo phenomenon was a new one on me. So the pink elephant and the pink bow have a little black dot each to keep the numbers even. That makes me happy – I'm a Libra, which is the scales of balance!

My radiation began four days later. The actual treatment involved lying on a massage-type table except the surface was rock hard, with a small flying saucer on a huge arm above me. There were no tunnels, needles, gas chambers or scary sore instruments. Because my target area was my neck, I had a bird's eye view of the flying saucer in action. The disc is about the same size as a small satellite dish. The part that points towards the area to be treated is covered in glass. Under the glass I could see a row of black slides. If you can imagine a box of thicker-in-dimension After Eight chocolates, you have a radiation machine in your mind's eye. Not as tasty to eat but very effective in killing cancer cells. Instead of being gooey and minty, these After Eights emanate bright-green shards of laser light. The machine also sends out an image of numbers, all in a row, projecting a ruler onto the skin. This ruler and its measurement numbers are the guide the radiologist needs to work out the exact positioning of the radiation rays.

A round of number-calling ensued, as two radiology nurses took control.

'Move fifteen to the left, ninety-three, three bags full …' And other such jargon, which they seemed to understand.

'OK, Emma, you just stay still. You can breathe away as normal.' There's a lot of holding your breath in a CT scan, so she wasn't being odd in mentioning that fact. 'We'll be back shortly.'

They left the room and I lay on the bed in the large room, with the bright-green laser show. Some clicking noises came from the flying saucer as the things that looked exactly like an old-fashioned slide show moved around a bit. Then a high-pitched but not loud noise.

Almost immediately, the radiologists trooped back into the room.

'That's it for today. Well done, Emma.' They helped me down from the massage-type table.

Now, maybe you know more than I do about radiation – which wouldn't be hard. I was utterly baffled as to how a minute-long session of microwaving my neck was going to kill any lingering bastard cancer cells.

I went a full week of trotting in and out, smiling and acting like it was all normal, before I broke cover and asked fifty questions all in a row. Like a human machine gun. 'I know you do this all the time and you're busy. I can tell by the way you buzz in and out of here that it's run-of-the-mill to you, but I'm having a total block with my brain connecting on all of this. Can you attempt to explain, in preschool language, how a minute of apparently nothing once a day kills cancer?'

'Well, your cells take twenty-four hours to recreate themselves. Radiation kills the bad ones and spares the good ones. So we keep up the destruction of the nasty ones every twenty-four hours for a few weeks, like a constant onslaught. The radiation builds up in your system until it finally peaks by the end of the relevant number of sessions. What's amazing is that the radiation continues to work for up to four weeks afterwards. So not only does it work with the here and now, but it also provides lasting protection after the fractions finish.'

'Stunning. I still don't really understand the ins and outs of the radiation concept, but that's fine, as I don't have to do it on myself or anyone else for that matter.' I nodded in awe.

I chose to trust the radiology team, who knew all the right buttons to push on the computer and how long to fry each person for. It was one of those situations where I narrowed my eyes and stroked my chin, frowning to look intelligent, and tried with all my might not to look as stupid as I felt. Clear as mud, between you and me.

OK, I get the killing the bad cells lark, but after that … Flying saucer … Sun-bed-type burn … Tiredness … Who? What? How the hell? I desperately wanted to ask how in the name of God they even found out that this sort of controlled frying worked in the first place. But a sixth sense screamed at me just to let it go.

Step away from the flying saucer, Emma. Your life won't stop just because you can't grasp the concept of radiation and its connection with the end of cancer.

My skin reacted mildly by turning pink and becoming itchy on the area around the scar and at the exit point in my back. It did its work on the site and left out the back. I felt a little more tired than usual during treatment but it was a walk in the park in comparison to chemotherapy.

The feeling when a course of treatment is finally finished is beyond wonderful. When a new course of radiation or chemotherapy begins, I always have a strong sense of determination and a dogged approach, which makes me drop-kick the first couple of sessions. It's usually by the time I'm a third of the way through that the reality of the situation hits me: I'm not yet halfway there so it's not a proper milestone, and there's still a way to go before the light at the end of the tunnel. God knows where it comes from, but a second burst of strength tends to explode like a phoenix from the ashes, and my body and mind just go where I need them to go.

The end of a round of treatment brings on a wonderful feeling of euphoria. It's both exciting and a relief and brings with it an unquenchable sense of optimism. And, as I've said before, there's a deep-rooted sense of pride. I know I had no choice with regard to my treatment. I could either go ahead with it, and hope for the right outcome, or refuse treatment and put myself on Death Row. But the feeling of accomplishment at the end is almost worth having cancer for! Almost …

Chapter 40

The Victory Dance

Score so far: Cancer 0: Emma 3. Cue the victory dance once more.

It was December 2009 and I had done it again. I had beaten cancer for the third time.

We like it a lot. Oh, yes. So – cue the bluebirds and the lovely Disney music? 'Surely now it's time,' I hear you cry!

Yep, you're forgiven for thinking I must have had enough at that stage. If I'm truthful, I felt nearer to closure on the whole cancer journey than I had before. I kind of hoped I'd earned my stripes. But guess what? Yes, sir. Yes, ma'am. I wasn't finished just yet.

My new career had taken off. I was writing full-time and loving it. The children were getting bigger by the second and more fun to be with than ever before. Cian was still being a triathlon bunny and working away in the flailing business world. We survived the recession. We all survived my cancer three times in as many years.

When I say 'we', I mean my family, friends and myself. Cancer doesn't affect just the patient. It hits all those in its immediate radius. Yes, I was the one who withstood the treatment and drugs, but each and every one of the people I know and love shared the hit. We all took the battering. We all shared the worry. We all wished, hoped and, if it was a personal preference, prayed that I would recover. Because I spoke out and, perhaps selfishly, spread my burden around, it meant that 'we' had beaten cancer for the third time.

I probably sound like a broken record – although that reveals my age! I ought to be a scratched CD or even a virus-riddled iPod or a wonky memory stick to be relevant today. I cannot stress just how much I believe in talking. I don't mean do a Shirley Valentine and talk to the wall. Talk to family, friends, your pet cat, even sit on park benches and prey on unsuspecting strangers. Whatever it takes. Go to a professionally trained counsellor or cancer support group if that rocks your boat. But promise me you won't sit in silence. Promise you won't bottle it up and let the cancer silence you. I am adamant that allowing sickness or troubles to take your voice is more damaging than the physical ailment.

I was born with the gift of the gab. I chat to people of all ages and cultures. I am a people-person. I enjoy my alone time in limited amounts. I absolutely adore writing, which is obviously a solitary thing. But at the end of the day, I know I would shrivel up and die if I had nobody to talk to.

If you are the type of person who would rather gouge your own eye out with a spoon than talk about your inner thoughts, try writing them down. But I would urge you to get the feelings out there. Place your trust in others, and I would be astonished if you don't reap the rewards. Each time I get the all-clear, I send another of my texts. The joyous ones are obviously much easier to word than the nasty ones with more bad news. But that whole notion of having to know pain to know joy is so true. Each time I get the all-clear, I have this slamming realisation of what it is to be healthy. I have another defining moment when I am grounded and have that crazy out-of-body experience when I know I am only a dot on this planet – yet I'm a happy and healthy dot.

In May 2010, I knew I wasn't feeling quite right. I'd been dragging myself around, knowing my energy levels were too low for comfort. I'd had almost five months of feeling a lot stronger and now, suddenly, I was under par again. The euphoria had faded goodo.

My head began to itch. The rash was coming back. Like a woman crossed with a chimp, I poked and prodded, rooted and scratched. Bingo – I found three more rubber peas. This time, for the first time ever, they were on the right side of my neck rather than the left. Jumping into action, I landed in Blackrock Clinic yet again.

Dr Fennelly issued a PET scan. Once again I played the waiting game. This time, more than any other, I was utterly paralysed by fear.

Because the cancer had moved to the right side of my body for the first time, I feared the very worst. I somehow figured that it must have stopped off in several organs on the way across from the left side.

With female logic, I decided it would have packed enough bags to see it through a fairly decent holiday. What's the point in going from Ireland to Australia for a weekend? None. You'd go for at least three weeks, wouldn't you? Well, being slightly left of centre in my thinking on most subjects, I figured cancer would apply similar logic. If it was going to jump out of its comfort zone – on the left side of my body – and journey to the right side, it had probably packed a large suitcase of bastard cells to deposit on the way. My biggest worry was which route it had taken. Had it gone straight across the main motorway, the direct line of lymph nodes across my chest, or by the scenic route? There were so many options open to the cancer: had it finally decided to stop off in my lungs, liver and perhaps taken in a kidney for the extra experience? Even worse, had it headed for the hills, looking for a high-altitude experience, and travelled via my brain? That made me think of the bits connected to my brain, such as my spine.

The last three times the cancer had been contained. Maybe my luck was running out. I had noticed I was breathless after climbing stairs. I had a heavy feeling in my chest too. I was convinced my lungs were infected, and God knew what other bits of me.

I actually thought I was toast. For the first time since the beginning of my journey, I felt like I was starting to drown. I wasn't so sure I would be able to beat this attack.

Six days passed between the PET scan and my much anticipated phone call from Dr Fennelly – six slow, torturous days, when the hours seemed to go on forever. I spent the nights tossing and turning, as I willed my mind to stop whirring. I scolded myself if I allowed my brain to go off on a what-if tangent. But, believe me, it's not easy to keep yourself on the reality track when you feel like a runaway train with no driver at the helm. I took sleeping tablets, but my own imagination was like an override button. Nothing allowed me to switch off. I conducted my days in as normal a manner as I could. I went through the motions and did all the things that were required of me. I dropped the children to school, made myself go swimming, bought groceries, did my writing, cooked dinner, washed and ironed clothes. All of it was on autopilot, as I tried to quash the taunting inner voice I was attempting to ignore.

What if I'm riddled with cancer this time? What if it's been on a record-breaking dash through my entire body? What if I have only two weeks to live?

When David Fennelly rang to tell me my organs were clear, I felt like I'd won the lottery. I felt giddy with relief. I had seconds of delight followed by a need to pinch myself in case I was dreaming.

'But what about the weird heavy feeling in my chest? Are my lungs clear?' I was almost afraid to ask.

'There are some tiny infected nodes in your upper chest, but your lungs are fine, Emma.'

I felt like running up the middle of the M50, shouting at the oncoming traffic: 'I'm not rampant with disease. I'm going to survive!' But as I was in line for another battle and I'd managed to stay alive that far, I figured playing chicken with rush-hour traffic on a very fast and busy motorway might be a bit of a waste. Let's face it, having 'She beat cancer three times and jumped in front of a Fiat 500' on my gravestone might make passers-by grin, but it would be a right pisser, wouldn't it?

Instead I listened to what Dr Fennelly had in mind for the latest round of my fight. The brawl had begun once again.

The fight plan this time would involve more radiation under the watchful eye of Dr Moriarty. This man is one of life's true gentlemen. He is gentle, serene and he instils confidence in the most gorgeous way imaginable. There was no hardship involved in returning to St Vincent's to see him again.

I had ten fractures of radiation to my neck, to melt and kill the infected nodes. The nodes (known to you and me as rubber peas) were growing by the minute. In the beginning I only found two: by the time I started radiation two weeks later, there were four. They seemed to be multiplying at a rate of knots.

Due to the other little buggers in my chest, Dr Fennelly wanted me to have more chemotherapy. My heart sank. I'd suffered so many infections and lost so much energy on chemotherapy before, and if

I'm honest, I wasn't sure I could take any more. But the news was good. I could take the chemotherapy in tablet form. My veins were to be spared and Percy the port need not be put back – praise the Lord! Called Xeloda, the tablets would be taken in two-week cycles. I would take two tablets twice daily for two weeks. Then I'd have a tablet-free week before repeating the cycle.

'You've to take them for six months and we'll review the situation then with scans,' Dr Fennelly explained.

The fear of going down the whole wig, port, sickness and infection route had made me think I didn't want more chemotherapy. But now that I knew my hair would remain and I wouldn't have burst veins, I was actually relieved to know I would have the added cover of the drug. I hoped that the simultaneous administration of both therapies at once might knock the cancer finally on the head.

Xeloda, as well as being a cancer killer, serves as a little highlighter for the radiation machine. It basically helps the radiation rays to batter the cancer cells properly. I was delighted to be able to use it. As far as side effects were concerned, this was meant to be much less invasive than the intravenous doses. It wouldn't cause alopecia. When I lost my hair, I honestly didn't give a toss. It was such a minor part of the bigger picture. But now that I'd been there and done that, I wasn't so keen to go back. Besides, I'd just paid to have my colour done. We all want to stretch each highlight job for as long as possible, so I was in no mood for being bald again.

The nausea wasn't meant to be as bad. The effect on Phil, my friendly white blood cells friend, was alleged to be less harsh. So, all in all, this drug was bad news for cancer, but much better news for the patient. Bring it on!

The radiation went smoothly and Dr Moriarty was pleased with my reaction. My skin became slightly red, but nothing more. However, the tiredness that enveloped me this time around was flooring. I have never known fatigue like it. The only comparison I can put my finger on is that feeling, after a few drinks, when you wake from a dream about going to the toilet. Jolting out of bed, you realise your bladder is about to burst so you stagger to the bathroom. You misjudge the door frame and bash your shoulder, nearly dislocating it, then stub your toe on an abandoned pair of shoes and finish off by whacking your elbow off the sharp bit of the shower door. When you finally plonk onto the toilet seat … That feeling of knackered, dazed, slightly chilly discomfort? Hold it for an entire day and you've just stepped into the world of radiation at its worst. Not life-threatening and not as bad as a really violent dose of the trots or an ear infection, when you feel like you've a hot needle in your brain, but not entirely pleasant either.

But, as with most things both good and bad, the middle-of-the-night dazed sensation and the radiation both passed. The chemotherapy was well under way and I was tolerating it with apparent ease. I went on my previously planned holiday to Spain with my friends Bernie, Ruth and Karen and our respective offspring. Between us we had enough children to start our own school! We soaked up the sun – well, I sat like a bat in a cave under an umbrella with duffel-coat-strength sunscreen on. My skin is blue at the best of times, but the Xeloda tablets require minimal sun exposure, so my answer was to apply fake tan at night instead. We swam, ate, drank, ate, shopped, ate and did some more eating. I don't know about you, but this idea of sunshine making people too hot to eat doesn't ever work for me. I eat ten times the usual amount. I also have a fascination with foreign supermarkets and buy trolley loads of stuff because it looks different. I will sit and eat packets of biscuits that taste like Styrofoam with fake chocolate flavouring in the middle, just because they're there. But that's what holidays are all about, and we enjoyed the time away.

Being on chemotherapy didn't disturb my two weeks of bliss and I didn't feel like a cancer carrier. On previous breaks, I'd ended up in awful rat holes with infections and I was grateful that didn't happen in Spain.

Needless to say, it couldn't all be plain sailing. I returned on a Wednesday night in the wee hours of the morning and was back in Blackrock Clinic for Avastin the following afternoon only to discover I had low blood counts and an infection. But that was a small price to pay for two weeks of fun.

However, while we were in Spain I had noticed a small lump forming under my left ear. It had felt like a marble at first. Then I thought it was one of those glands at the top of your neck beside the jaw that the doctor always checks when you say you've got a sore throat.

But the marble grew. So I pointed it out to the nurses while I was in the hospital.

I wasn't feeling too panicked, as I was already taking my chemotherapy. I knew I was doing all the right things. My main concern was that it wasn't a whole new batch of cancer, one that had manifested in spite of the recent radiation and ongoing chemotherapy. If it was an entirely new beast, flourishing and laughing in the face of the treatment, that would be scary.

A swift fumble in my neck and a nod to confirm it was an infected node was all I needed. Dr Moriarty was called upon again. He was kind and reassuring and explained that my previous PET scans had shown signs of activity in that area, but as no nodes were infected, they had chosen not to irradiate the area. 'Now that it's raised itself, we'll give it a single dose of radiation. That'll sort it for you, love,' he said kindly.

'Phew,' I said. 'I was terrified it might have been a new bout that you hadn't known about.'

'No, love, we knew that was there, so it's nothing we can't handle. You don't worry about it – I'll have it sorted in a jiffy,' he promised. Once again I had the planning CT scan, where the doctor and radiologist measured the size and depth of the infected node and planned the exact position of the radiation machine. I was still taking my chemotherapy, which Dr Moriarty explained previously worked as both a cancer slayer and highlighting substance. In other words, it would make the cancerous node stand out, thus presenting it in all its glory to the rays of radiation, making it ripe for zapping.

All the previous fractions had been done on a daily basis for approximately fifty seconds a pop. This different type of radiation called for a single zap, which lasted six minutes. Instead of the flying-saucer part of the machine hovering away from the affected area, this time the glass was flush up against my skin. There was no heat or sensation from the rays. Once again there was the faint high-pitched noise and bright lights, but that was all.

What I wasn't prepared for was the aftermath. I was perfect immediately afterwards. I went for a delicious lunch with my darling agent

Sheila. We scoffed sweet garlicky prawns and shared a dish of chocolate soup – yes, it was created and produced by angels. Utterly
divine.

We parted company, I drove home – and by the time I got inside
the house I felt like I'd been run over by a juggernaut. My face
swelled, my neck looked as if it belonged to a professional rugby
player and I felt pain so severe it was like I'd been kicked in the jaw
with a steel-capped boot. For the next two days, I was in bed, barely
able to move. I felt appalling, no two ways about it, but in my own
warped way it was quite satisfying. I kept reminding myself that it
was good that I felt so bloody dreadful – if the treatment was having
such a drastic effect on me, imagine what it was doing to the cancer.

Slowly over the next week the sickly tiredness, which was akin
to morning sickness at its worst, ebbed away. I still didn't feel quite
right, though. By now, dear reader, you're probably thinking – enough
already. But, my sixth sense didn't let me down. I had another few
nodes festering and forming. Just up from the previous marble, two
other smaller marbles came to stay. I'd had a pain in my inner ear
and often, for no apparent reason, a swishing noise would drift into
play. As before, I plagued St David Fennelly. (I've decided he needs
to be promoted from doctor to saint.) Another meeting was set up
with St Michael Moriarty (he too needs to evolve to sainthood in
my eyes). The usual predictive scan took place and the nodes were
pinpointed.

Once again the treatment was to involve the single dose, the
whamming mallet of radiation. This time I was ready and armed
with drugs! I organised for the children to be entertained by willing
and loyal family and friends, and made sure there were fresh, clean
sheets on the bed and plenty of Difene at the ready.

Perhaps it was a case of been-here-before-got-the-T-shirt, but the
second blast didn't floor me quite as much as the previous one.
Knowing what's coming is a great advantage. I firmly believe that
having an idea of what to expect removes at least half of the pain
and stress of treatment. It was like I'd physically and mentally (not
to mention chemically, with pain relief tablets) built up my own
armour. I pitched up with my virtual sword and lay on the radiation
table saying to myself, 'Bring it on.'

I found the next few weeks a struggle. I was so toxic from the three-way hit of chemotherapy tablets, intravenous Avastin and radiation, my bowel decided to play dead. I think it actually closed its eyes and put its fingers in its ears and refused to function. As a result I went around with a tummy like a pregnant person for six days. I was so bloated and felt so vile, I considered buying a maternity dress. I even eyed up one of our king-sized duvet covers, wondering if I could get away with wearing it as a dress. Perhaps if I teamed it with a cool pair of boots and some jazzy accessories, people might think it was one of those eccentric couture pieces?

Instead I rang the clever and wonderful angels, otherwise known as oncology nurses, in Blackrock Clinic and they prescribed a course of industrial bowel unblocking potions.

Between May and October of 2010 I'd had to find and deal with three spots of cancer. If the notion of all things coming in groups of three is gospel, then surely I was due a break, for a while at least?

Obviously, I was growing increasingly weary of having cancer, again and again. If given the choice, I would have loved to draw a line in the sand at that point, loved to never have a reoccurrence. But as cancer doesn't offer a multiple-choice menu of possibilities, I would have to keep my sword sharpened. If cancer did strike again, I would continue to fight. I'd come way too far to even consider backing down.

Chapter 41

It's Cancer v Emma Once More!

I got a couple of months' grace. Time to recharge my batteries, write another book and jump back into life. By life I mean going out past nine o'clock at night, having the odd glass of wine and leading a non-medical existence. I grabbed it with both hands. I wrote my third novel, *The Pink Ladies Club*, and revelled in the freedom from all things cancerous.

I know a small part of me genuinely believed that I would stay well. I don't regret thinking that – in fact, I know it's part of the reason I've stayed sane this long. Hope is a wonderful thing and without it life would be pretty miserable.

Six months into 2011 I began to feel my body slowing down. I also began to put on weight for no reason. I hadn't started eating all the pies, yet I was beginning to morph into Emma in a fat suit. I knew before the lumps appeared that the cancer was back.

This time it went hell for leather. I had tumours on both sides of my neck in several places and it seemed to be growing by the minute right in front of my eyes.

I waited with nail-biting trepidation as the scan results were processed.

Knowing this latest bout needed to be stopped in its tracks, David Fennelly ordered my old friend chemotherapy to come into the ring. The fight was on once again.

Taxol was the poison of choice and I was warned it might have some harsh side effects, the first of which was that I would lose my hair. The treatment was weekly for the first twelve weeks, moving to two weekly after that. Could I bear to use the scalp cooler for that frequency? I thought long and hard about it and figured the exorbitant amount of money I'd literally just shelled out for highlights at the hairdresser's was a good enough reason on its own for saving my honeyed tresses.

I wasn't especially worried about losing my hair for my own sake. It was more for the children. They were ten and eleven respectively and were far more aware of the potential dangers of cancer. If I could avoid looking like a victim, I was going to do it.

I took Valium before each session and hoped I would be able to endure the freezing helmet. In the years since I'd first tried the scalp cooler things had moved on. The cap looked neater and slightly less uncomfortable.

So I pitched up at Blackrock Clinic and lovely Riza lathered my dry hair in conditioner. Apparently the creamy liquid works fabulously to stop the icy cap sticking to the hair and thus pulling it out at the end of the treatment.

That first morning, when the ice-dripping, tight-fitting helmet was pulled onto my head, it made me want to sob like a baby. The intensity of how astonishingly freezing it feels is difficult to put into words. It took my breath away. It made me talk in shunting gasps as I attempted to assure Riza that I was OK and could cope. Painkillers and a tablet of fuzziness to make the world a little floaty and help me 'relax' didn't seem to help one jot. But having said that, I did manage to stop myself from cursing like a sailor or indeed doing open-mouthed ugly crying. So perhaps it did help a little.

I'd be lying if I said I found the cold cap easy to withstand. I am a cold-blooded creature at the best of times. Any of my friends will confirm that our house is always like a sauna. I feel the cold like nobody else I know. So this wasn't exactly my idea of fun. But enduring the cold became my new-found battle. It was something to concentrate on and something to be utterly dogged about.

Once the initial ten minutes passed, and my entire skull became one with the frozen helmet, things improved. Well, improved is probably a loose term but I guess I was sufficiently numbed that the panting and involuntary gasping could cease. Randomly, globs of ice would melt and drop down my back. It was essentially like sitting under a dribbling bucket of ice. But I kept thinking of my hair and how losing it all, yet again, wasn't really up there with the things I wanted to do.

So I persevered that first day. Riza brought me heat packs – so many that I was the closest thing to a boiler with a handmade lagging jacket imaginable. The thin, cardboard-like hospital blankets did little to ward off the cold, but the nurses wrapped me in as many as they could. The cold seeped from my head to my extremities. My lips turned an unusual shade of violet and my fingers paled to a milky corpse-like shade. They also decided they weren't going to function any longer, admitting defeat to the unwanted cold, so I was handed umpteen cups of boiling water to cradle! My feet, once they decided to do an impression of a plastic mannequin's, became blocky as they sent horrid little shivers of cold up my quivering calves.

On the upside (I sat for an hour prior to the administration of the chemotherapy – to ensure my head and follicles were truly frozen), once the chemotherapy was started I wouldn't have cared if they'd put arsenic in the drip! I was given Taxol first, followed by Avastin and some fluids in between. That was a doddle. The deal with the scalp cooler is that I had to keep it on for two hours after the chemotherapy drip finished. It's held in place by a tight-fitting strap that goes under the chin, and once I was vaguely immune to the cold, the strap took over as public enemy number one. The clenching tightness under my jaw, and thus the pressure on the hinge joints on either side, was pretty dreadful. I'd be lying if I said it became comfortable or that I simply forgot I was wearing a Baltic snowball.

It was almost worth having the scalp cooler on for those hours to experience the relief of having it removed. That moment was blissful. I had fanfares going off in my head, and the feeling of normal air as it kissed my slightly crusty frozen hair was wonderful. The helmet is attached to a large corrugated tube, making it pretty heavy too. So I actually felt as if I might float around the room like a tiny feather on a breeze. Maybe the relaxant tablet had worked really well after all …

Riza in the Oncology unit was at pains to point out that the scalp cooler would only preserve my hair if I looked after it. That meant treating it with kid gloves. No excessive brushing, washing it once a week (prior to this I washed my hair every day!) and no heat products such as a hair dryer or straightener. I followed her instructions to the last detail. The effort worked and, although my hair thinned considerably, I didn't lose it all. I also had my shoulder-length hair cut to a lighter and easier-to-manage chin length.

By this time my veins were struggling to cope with yet more drugs being flushed through them. I actually felt bad for the phlebotomists as they tried (always with a smile, bless them) to access my ever-flattening veins.

I knew the time was coming when I'd need another port. My first one was a horrible yoke and I resisted until my arms looked like those of a heroin addict. I was bruised, sore and utterly miserable, so I finally relented. I cannot express how glad I was to have my second port inserted. Like everything else I was experiencing, ports had come on hugely too. Gone was the hard metal and instead I was given one called a Dignity port. It did as its name suggested and offered me shed-loads of dignity. It's still visible under my skin, but for some reason I don't view it with the same hate as its predecessor. The relief at not having my poor arms stabbed was worth the pain.

It was put in on a Friday morning by a lovely heart surgeon. I convinced him to allow me to remain awake during the procedure. So, with local anaesthetic, he got to work.

'Could you turn the screen around, please?' I asked. 'I can't see what you're doing.'

Apparently that was the intention, but Mr Brophy kindly obliged and allowed me to watch his work on my own personal live television! I had a rather lumpy and messy-looking scar from where Percy had once resided, so he kindly tidied that up at the same time.

The following morning I was bruised in every colour of the rainbow – think black eye but at the top of the chest. Nasty looking for a spell, but oh so worth it in the end.

To this day I still can't say I love the moment the nurses access my port. It involves a little bit of prodding followed by a piercing of the skin, as a rather large needle is pushed into it, but I know it's the lesser of two evils. It's a very short, sharp pop and pinch and that's it over and done with. My arms are normal looking and I no longer have that burning, throbbing sensation as the bruises struggle to heal.

For a couple of years I had a bit of an icky feeling when I looked in the mirror and saw the small tube under my skin that leads from the port directly into my jugular vein. It made me squint my eyes and stick out my tongue in an involuntary manner.

I also shopped to hide it. Silly as it might sound, I went through a period of at least two years where I wouldn't wear clothes that showed off the port. I was convinced that people would hone in on it and react the way I did, with the sticky-out tongue and squinty eyes, like they'd sucked a lemon. But as the years have passed I've come to care less about it. In fact, I've probably come to the correct conclusion that other people aren't actually that interested in my port or any other minute detail on my body! As my grandmother often used to tell us grandchildren if we had a pimple on our faces as teenagers – nobody is looking at you that closely. I think she had a point!

The effects of the Taxol and Avastin cocktail were nowhere near as dreadful as I'd anticipated. Although I felt that familiar crawling-under-my-skin sensation, I wasn't a nauseous mess. The best part was that I began to feel better almost instantly, cancer-wise. By my fourth treatment I was seeing the difference. The hardened and growing lumps were beginning to soften around the edges and diminish. My real battle, if there was one, was with the endurance test that was the scalp cooler.

As I write this I wonder what possessed me to continue with it. It was so unpleasant and I began to dream about being stuck on an iceberg or, one night, being run over by the *Titanic* as I slept. But once the number of treatments began to clock up and I knew I was sailing forth, it would've been a real shame to waste all that freezing and give in.

For me, the scalp cooler preserved most of my hair. It was still incredibly fragile, though. I could only wash it if I really needed to – if I was going on TV or out in public where I couldn't have lank-looking strings on my head, with a distracting hairband or clip-on head piece. I made friends with dry shampoo too. This stuff varies in price, and now lots of types, from the Kardashians' to own-brand versions, are on offer. For my purposes, the bog-standard one by Batiste that has been on the market for aeons worked perfectly well. Another key to preserving my hair was minimal brushing. Obviously every time we brush our hair the odd few strands are going to come away. But during this time, it was as if I were brushing my hair with a sharp razor. The brush would get clogged with hair, making me want to shout at it in frustration.

So I moved from being a hair-wash-every-day gal to a twice-a-week version. It took me a while to get used to not washing my head in the shower each morning, but it was the only way I could hold on to enough hair to see me through.

Would I recommend the scalp cooler? In a word, yes. It's not for the faint-hearted or the cold-blooded, but I had mastered the art of staying warm by the time I came to the end of that chemotherapy cycle. I was given a present of a fabulous pair of duck-down-filled booties by a fellow patient, Fiona Tiernan. She'd discovered them and kindly bought me a pair.

They still remind me of her; sadly Fiona passed away.

For all the world they looked like boots made from a duvet, and they fit snugly over my three pairs of bed socks – the soft fluffy ones that come in a three-pack from Primark with the sticky bits on the soles. Then came the long johns from M&S under thick tracksuit bottoms. On top, I went with a stylish long-sleeved thermal skiing vest, also from M&S, with a polo neck and topped off with a cashmere jumper. Yes, that might sound a little arsey, but cashmere has the wondrous ability to make us warm without being bulky. I would've sold my shoe collection on eBay to afford one.

I also brought a Puffa coat, which I held off on putting on until I began to go numb. I've no doubt I looked like I had become homeless, with nowhere to store my clothing, so I'd simply put it all on. But believe me, there's not a lot of glamour going on in the Oncology unit, and being warm was of paramount importance. Besides, I didn't have to see myself. I will take this opportunity to apologise to anyone who had to look at me during that time. But I hope they might understand that style goes out the window when there's a snowball on your head for eight hours.

Meanwhile, sandwiched between doses of poison, I released my third novel, *Miss Conceived*. It was a bestseller in Ireland. Simultaneously, the first version of this very book hit the shelves. As a result I was catapulted onto the screens of RTÉ and TV3 in Ireland. I appeared on the *Late Late Show* to tell my story of being diagnosed and beating the odds. Next came *Ireland AM* and I was selected as a regular panellist on *Midday*, the all-women show. A whole new world opened up to me. I had always loved doing radio, and that didn't change, but live TV was another string to my bow that I hadn't ever anticipated. I loved it instantly and found it easy to speak about a subject that had been taboo for so many years in Ireland.

The tsunami of warmth and encouragement was astonishing, and as more and more cancer patients and non-cancer sufferers began to reach out to me, I was blown away. To this day, I receive countless messages from others who feel they can 'talk' to me, by email and even by snail mail. My postman is brilliant and has delivered umpteen letters with the simple address of 'Author Emma Hannigan, Bray, Co Wicklow'!

Through all of this, I know my writing kept me afloat. After all, what other job would allow me to work from a hospital bed or at home in my pyjamas or indeed with a snowball on my head?

My positivity never faded. I knew that there was so much more of my life to live. I knew that I was only getting going with my career and that there was still a plan in place for me. That may sound odd, especially as I don't follow any formal religion and nor am I what one might call God-fearing. But I knew in my heart that my time was far from up yet.

In late November of 2011 I got an unexpected call from my local town council offices. They asked if I would consider becoming an ambassador for Bray. I was thrilled. What a wonderful honour, and of course I was happy to agree. I didn't realise until I went along to the presentation that another person was being honoured that day too – Katie Taylor. My grandfather was a champion boxer and I have always had a keen interest in the sport, so Katie Taylor was right up there in the admiration stakes for me. I was nervous about meeting her and wasn't sure what to expect. She turned out to be the most humble and astonishingly special person. We formed an instant bond and I'm proud to call her my friend. We see one another as often as life allows and we're in constant contact on the phone. Since that time, Katie famously won a gold medal at the 2012 Olympics and is European and World champion umpteen times over. She is now making astonishing progress as a professional boxer. She inspires me and leads me to believe that women are capable of anything if they dare to dream and are prepared to work hard to achieve big goals. We need more women like Katie in this world.

The other happy news was that the chemotherapy had worked like a dream. All signs of the cancer disappeared. I escaped without any sleepovers at the hospital. I had a couple of knee-buckling and eye-wateringly uncomfortable urinary tract infections, but, hey, they're free with the treatment.

I read a clatter of books by alternative practitioners along with ones by medical doctors. There was a common thread in many of them, linking the intake of dairy products with cancer reoccurrence. So, with a heavy heart, I made the decision to cut all dairy from my diet.

It was hell. No chocolate! I didn't care about milk or cheese or butter. There are so many alternatives for those. But have you ever tasted dairy-free chocolate? If you haven't – don't. There's no substitute for chocolate in my book. I literally went on a diet of denial. That was how it felt.

After a few months of it, I really began to feel frustrated. I read the ingredients of every package of food, I ordered dairy-free dishes when we went out. In short, I'd become a food bore. I hated being that way. I love food and love enjoying meals out. But in the back of my mind I kept thinking that perhaps this denial would save me from getting cancer again. That would, of course, make it all worthwhile.

Meanwhile, my career continued to flourish. I signed to a new publisher and agreed to write two books the following year. Most authors do one a year, so I was pushing the boat out in every possible way. It felt great. It was my own way of raising two fingers to cancer and getting on with life in spite of what was happening.

By December I was finished my six months of treatment and was called in for scans. Drinking the Pernod-flavoured bottle of scan preparation wasn't any easier. In fact, I now dribble in disgust almost before I taste it. As usual I talked to my body (not out loud – I'd finished the treatment and couldn't risk being locked up for another six months) while the large gaping tunnel scanned my body for lingering traces of cancer.

Mercifully I got an early Christmas present of clear scans. Once again, I revelled in the euphoria of my wellness. I never have any idea how long the feeling will last before the cheeky cancer comes crashing back, so I celebrate each time. I go about with a goon-like smile and outsiders would be forgiven for thinking I'm slightly bonkers.

Once again I was hurtling towards my favourite time of the year filled with Christmas cheer!

For the second consecutive year we went *en famille* to Dromoland Castle to eat, drink and ring in the New Year. As I stood in my sparkly dress surrounded by the people I love the most, I felt palpably lucky, blessed and incredibly grateful to be alive.

I know each and every one of us has waves of poignant memories flood our senses on New Year's Eve. After all, that's exactly why many people dread and detest that night. But that year, as I observed a ballroom filled with jubilant revellers of all ages embracing and gravitating towards the dance floor to join hands and raise the roof with a raucous rendition of 'Auld Lang Syne', I felt as if my heart might burst with joy.

Chapter 42

A Day Without Chocolate Makes One Weak

Maybe I crossed my fingers correctly as I made a wish that New Year's Eve, maybe the angels got together and knitted me a little protective layer, but whatever the reason, 2012 became my first year since 2007 without cancer.

I rejoiced in the liberation of it all. Dr Fennelly kept me on a retainer dose of Avastin to protect my organs, but that was great because it offered me peace of mind and ensured I was being closely monitored.

Home life was the same as anyone else's in so far as my kids, who were hurtling towards their teenage years, found me unbearably embarrassing in every single way. I was satisfied with that and felt it was fitting and comfortingly 'normal'.

I had more energy than I ever remember having and felt ten years younger. I'd forgotten how it felt to be well and it was incredible. I was still on my dairy-free diet and still gazing longingly at bars of chocolate. I allowed myself a couple of squares of 85 per cent dark stuff every now and then. But I hated the waxy, slightly greasy texture, along with the bitter just-licked-an-ashtray aftertaste. I was friends with rice milk, almond milk and sunflower spread instead of butter. I cook all food from scratch so it wasn't ever an issue at home. It was just annoying when eating out.

I cleaned up my diet and made sure I was starting my day with porridge, seeds and manuka honey. I bought a juicer and became a juice pusher. The whole house was force-fed a fruit and vegetable juice every morning. They can be delicious if the right blend is used and I weaned Kim onto them by adding honey. I was swimming a few times a week and walking as often as I could. This may sound like a normal amount of exercise, but coming from an exercise-phobe like me, it was gargantuan!

Cian started his dream business. His obsession with triathlons hadn't dwindled over the years – in fact he'd become a trillion times worse. The entire country seemed to be gripped by the exercise bug too. He saw a gap in the market, along with having a genuine interest and desire to do a job he loved. Base2Race, his sports emporium, opened at the height of a global recession during the worst weather spell Ireland had seen for years. They had to dig the snow away from the doors on opening day! Working with a group of like-minded, ambitious colleagues, a new business and way of life was born. If it were possible to make this work, Cian, Dominic, Paul, Darren, Eanna and Damian would do it. They all put their hearts and souls into Base2Race and so far it's going from strength to strength, year on year. This is yet another example of positivity and belief overcoming the odds. If Cian had a euro for every time someone had told him he was insane opening a business during a recession, we'd be living on a tropical island with a huge retirement package by now!

Besides, as a couple, we figured we'd survived enough adversity to teach us how to remain upbeat about taking a chance. It proved to be a positive move in every possible way.

I continued to sit on the panel on *Midday* with my friend and host Elaine Crowley, where I met all sorts of women with a vast array of life experience. I wrote as if my life depended on it and signed a contract with Hachette Books Ireland. My editor Ciara Doorley (who edited this very tome) became my writing wing-woman, and together we produced my fourth novel, *Keeping Mum*. Through Ciara I learned more about writing than I had ever dreamed possible. So enthused was I by the whole process that I took off on a tangent and indulged one of my greatest loves – Christmas. I slipped into the deliciousness of writing a Christmas-themed novel. I love all things sparkly and twinkly. If I had my way I would have a Christmas tree in every room all year around. I love the family togetherness and the magic that Christmas brings. I've also been lucky enough to be able to enjoy this special time of year in the whole of my health so far. So I guess the joy and happiness this time of year evokes for me is sublime.

Hachette Ireland agreed to publish my second novel in one year, so in November 2012 *Driving Home for Christmas* hit the shelves. I loved promoting it and decided to drive around Ireland giving out home-baked mince pies to the booksellers as I signed copies! Ruth Shern from Hachette and I even donned flashing earrings and sparkly antlers at one point. We got some seriously odd looks – especially because it was only the beginning of November! But luckily Ruth is as enthused by all things sparkly as I am, so the strange looks or people walking into walls while staring at us didn't matter.

I'd managed a full year of being cancer free, and for the first time since I'd found out about the BRCA1 gene in 2005, I felt true hope that I had finally come to a point where I could leave the cancer trail in the distance.

The break was fantastic for my family too. Gone were the hospital appointments and the practicalities of having to juggle cancer with work and family life.

The relief was immense and I savoured each and every moment of that year. Not for one second did I take it for granted. Each morning that I woke cancer free was like a little prize. I still attended Blackrock Clinic for regular checks but nothing sinister seemed to be raising its ugly head. Hurray!

My career was slowly building as more new readers came on board and bought my books. I couldn't believe my luck at finding this incredible job surrounded by a team of people who believed in my work. My agent, Sheila Crowley, was excited and enthused by the reaction I was getting at home in Ireland and vowed to help me push things forward and bring my books to a wider audience. Things were on the up and I was pinching myself in delight!

That December a dear friend and fellow crazy lady, Britt Eccles, lost her fight with cancer. She left two beautiful children, Lucca and Sophie, an adoring husband, Colin, and heartbroken family and friends behind. Her funeral was lovely, if it's possible to say that. It was a humanist ceremony where people spoke about Britt and recalled stories of her short yet fun-filled life. Britt was a party girl who lived life to the full. I still struggle to believe a girl so beautiful, vivacious and endearing was taken away. Anyone who knew her will confirm that she had the loudest, most infectious laugh. When I close my eyes I can almost hear it. She and Colin had married in St Lucia in 1998. Cian and I had been there on our honeymoon so we had the privilege of being at the wedding. The unfairness and the injustice of Britt having to leave her two children and the wonderful life that she'd created has never left me. I think of her often and hope she is dancing among the stars, sipping champagne and throwing her head back, laughing in her distinctive way. She was one in a million and will never be forgotten.

Chapter 43

Survivor's Guilt

Tragedy struck again in September 2013 when my beloved uncle Neil passed away from his cancer. Leaving his beautiful wife and three daughters devastated, he finally found peace and his pain ended. He had fought for years but sadly his cancer had spread and raged out of control. He was forty-nine.

Yet again I was reminded of how lucky I am. Although my cancer seems to like returning, I am so grateful the treatments can eradicate it.

Although we didn't see one another that often, Neil and I used to converse over email – usually from one hospital to another. He had a dry and very dark sense of humour and we'd make each other giggle as we shared stories from the oncology wards. The day before he died I sat with him and held his hand. I told him he was a hero, which is the truth. He'd given the fight his all, but in the end the mountain was simply too high for anyone to climb. At his funeral I felt immense guilt that he hadn't made it but I had. It's drastically unfair but I am humbled and grateful to have survived this long.

I think of him and Britt all the time and wonder how they're getting on in heaven. I hope they've met up and shared a drink and a giggle.

My own health euphoria, coupled with my survivor's guilt, lasted until October 2013. Literally a month after Neil died the warning flag was raised as I began to feel exhausted. My scalp became itchy and I could sense a familiar stiffness in my limbs again. The honeymoon period was over and I could feel pressure and a dull, aching pain starting at the back of my skull. Within weeks my worst fears were realised as a lump began to form on the left external occipital crest – or, in plain English, at the base of my head where the skull meets the spine. This lump scared the bejaysus out of me. It was too close to that gooey grey matter and I honestly feared it was going to either spread in there to my brain or down my spine. It felt as hard as a rock and I wasn't prepared for a massive tumour on my head. As if it were attempting to collect a group of friends in order to make the most of the invasion, the cancer decided to form further tumours on both sides of my neck. This time they went for a mass gathering. So I ended up with several spectacularly impressive-looking bastards. Yes, they were visible to the human eye and, my word, they were ugly and instilled fear in everyone who saw them.

This time David Fennelly decided they should be fried, rather than having more chemotherapy. Darling Dr Moriarty had retired so I asked to see Professor John Armstrong at St Vincent's Private Hospital in Dublin.

I had been asked to speak at a radiation conference in Dublin's Croke Park during 2012 and the speaker after me happened to be Professor Armstrong. I'd never heard a more passionate and informed speech and left that day vowing that I would ask for him should the need ever arise.

Professor Armstrong is a different personality type to Dr Moriarty. The former was of the hand-holding and gently-does-it persuasion, whereas Professor Armstrong is more pragmatic and quite frankly announced to me that he didn't do small talk.

That's just fine by me. I knew this man was at the top of his game and I wasn't in the market for a new furry friend. In fact, at that scary time I sincerely needed someone to take charge of the monster that was threatening to cover my entire skull and eat me up from the inside out.

A long and arduous MRI scan was the first port of call. Even though I'd had CT scans and an ultrasound, that wasn't going to cut the mustard.

Professor Armstrong needed an MRI scan so he could plan the radiotherapy properly. Normally I'm fine with scans, but this time, as I lay on the table and inserted my yellow squidgy ear plugs and waited for the loud knocking noise, pain shot through my skull.

The hard surface of the table was leaving no leeway for the tumour on the back of my head. The weight of my head meant it was being squashed. It didn't like that one bit and let me know. The pain built and built until I felt as if I couldn't endure it one second longer.

When an MRI is happening the nurse always hands the patient a small buzzer. The idea is that you can press it at any time and the procedure will be halted.

I longed to press that button. I wanted nothing more than to stop the pain. But the voice inside my head stopped me. Professor Armstrong needed the images to plan my treatment. Without the treatment I wouldn't be in a very happy place. The cancer couldn't be encouraged to continue rampaging through my head and neck. This was the beginning of the end for the cancer: I simply had to endure it.

I got through the pain by saying the alphabet backwards and trying to recite the words of songs from the eighties. That made me dig deep into the recesses of my mind. I might have been in agony but a tiny part of me was also quite smug to realise that I knew many of the early Prince tracks off by heart all those years later.

What felt like a decade later, the knocking noise stopped. The nurse announced on loudspeaker that she was on her way in to release me.

I don't think I managed to have a proper conversation, not even a surfacey one about the weather. I staggered in my hospital gown to the changing cubicle and pulled my clothes back on. Bile rose in my throat and my head throbbed so violently that it was as if it had an angry alien trapped under the skin and it was flailing to get out.

My next port of call was for bloods. I sat like a dazed dolly and waited for my name to be called. At that moment they could've removed a limb and I wouldn't have cared.

Feeling ragged and shocked I went home and waited for a start date for the radiotherapy. I had no idea how many fractions I would need, but I'd decided it would probably be ten at the most. Nobody mentioned the number ten ever, but for some reason I felt that would be reasonable.

When the radiotherapy department got in touch, they warned me it would take three weeks to plan the procedure. I was glad that they were clearly taking their time and making sure the attention to detail was exact, but it also felt like a long wait. Meanwhile the tumours were growing so rapidly I felt I could video them and make my own David Attenborough-type movie. You know the ones where we see a flower changing from a tightly enclosed bud into a beautiful thing with splayed petals in fast forward? My version would be a head with a small bulge on the back that evolved into an elephant-woman-esque mass. Not exactly pleasant watching and I'm guessing nobody would actually want to see it.

Eventually, twenty years later – OK, two and a half weeks later – I got a call to say my treatment would begin the following Wednesday, 13 November.

As there was so much disease present, the treatment needed to be done in two halves. The left side with the elephant-woman mass on the skull was up first. I was slightly shocked to learn I'd need fifty fractions in total. Twenty-five on each side.

Professor Armstrong warned me that my salivary gland could be irreparably damaged. I would undoubtedly suffer with radiation burns to the skin and it was going to sap my energy.

While none of those things sounded like fun, I had no choice. The cancer had to be stopped before it took over. As before, a sense of dogged determination kicked in. I squared my shoulders, took a deep breath and promised myself I would give as good as I got.

I was called into St Vincent's to have a mask made. I'd never experienced this before, although I'd seen them many times at the hospital. They look, for all the world, like a plastic-mesh mummy in the shape of a head, neck and shoulders. My usual morbid fascination took over as I pitched up at the radiotherapy department. You know me, I love nothing more than nosing at something I've never had a go of before. Lovely Michelle was on hand to mould my mask. I lay on the CT scanning bed and she explained that she was going to drape a warmed plastic sheet over my face. She would grab this sheet at opposite sides and pull swiftly downward. My face and head would imprint in the pliable, hot plastic meshing and it would then harden quickly.

The purpose of the mask was to keep my head, neck and shoulders rigidly still while the machine was doing its zapping. If I moved or shunted while the radiotherapy was happening I'd be in danger of two things: first, missing the cancer, and second, damaging vital parts of my body, like my brain or throat, or other areas that wouldn't take kindly to being cooked.

Once the mask was set Michelle lifted it off. It was bizarre to see an imprint of my own head and shoulders. I skipped off home and readied myself for the course of radiotherapy. I had my printout with all the times. The machine runs from Monday to Friday, so I was in line for six weeks of toing and froing. The first half of treatment was scheduled to finish on 17 December, all going well. I'd have a few weeks off for good behaviour and Professor Armstrong would see me, assess how effective the treatment had been and, all things being equal, I'd have the second half of treatment early in the new year.

So If I thought the MRI scan was a low point, I was sorely mistaken. I've heard it said that when people experience true pain they hit rock bottom. Well it was as if the devil had watched the MRI procedure and chortled while holding his tummy and vowed to get a JCB to dig far deeper into the reservoir of pain. What followed was nothing short of torture, but before I go into that, I need to assure you that things weren't totally pants at that time.

As is the pattern in my life, it wasn't all about cancer and pain with me. On 9 November, just before I was scheduled to begin my treatment, I was nominated for an *Irish Tatler* magazine Women of the Year Award. I knew it would be one of Norah Casey's sublimely planned events with lots of sparkle and no expense spared. I was thrilled to be nominated, but didn't think for one second that I'd win.

Cian and I donned our black-tie gear and headed for Dublin's Four Seasons hotel. The bubbly was flowing and the style was astounding. We had our photo taken on the red carpet and milled around happily chatting to lots of other excited punters.

My agent, Sheila, joined us just as dinner began. The awards were beautifully presented. Norah didn't read out the lists of nominees followed by the winners – instead she only called the winning name, avoiding that awful moment where several people have to plaster a frozen smile on their faces as they hide their embarrassment or disappointment.

My category was the prestigious Literature Prize. Previous winners included authors such as Marian Keyes, Cathy Kelly, Anne Enright and Edna O'Brien so I was over the moon to be in the pot in the first place.

I almost fell off my chair when my name came up, followed by a VT of snippets of TV appearances with the covers of my books zooming wonderfully in and out! This was my first award for literature and to know that my work had resonated with the judging panel at *Irish Tatler* made me want to burst with pride. A job that was my saviour and my therapy and literally kept me afloat during the hard times was starting to shine more light on the darkness than I had ever anticipated. I still get a lump in my throat (a non-cancerous one – purely an emotional one, you understand!) when I think of that evening. It meant more than Norah Casey and the staff of *Irish Tatler* will ever know.

The following Wednesday, 13 November 2013, marked the start of my race against cancer diagnosis number nine. My first fraction wasn't until 4.30 in the afternoon, so I dropped the children to school and went into my office as normal. St Vincent's Hospital, where I needed to attend, is in the hub of south Dublin's traffic. Morning, noon and night this area is gridlocked, so I knew I needed to allow at least an hour to get there and the same to return to Bray. I tried not to stress about it, but I knew this process in all reality was going to take a minimum of three hours a day. I know it sounds a bit trivial to meow about giving up three hours a day – after all, the alternative was to continue growing a boulder on the back of my head and on both sides of my neck and to risk the cancer spreading and killing me. No contest. I know all that, but it was a pain in the neck – literally.

I pitched up that first day full of hope that my new mask and I were going to get along famously. Many of the radiotherapists I'd met before were still there, so there were plenty of familiar, smiling faces. But the second the mask was secured to the radiotherapy table all mirth and fun dissolved.

'I don't think I can stand the pain,' I struggled to say. The mask was so tight it made swallowing and talking difficult. I was clipped to the bed in several places, which made perfect sense. There was no wriggle room and therefore no room for error. I completely understood why it had to be so tight, but the pain was like nothing I have ever endured in my life.

The mass on my head had nowhere to go. It was the size of a tangerine, right on the edge of the occipital bone.

Professor Armstrong explained afterwards that the pain I was feeling was nerve pain. The cancer was just below the skin and pressed up against the bone of my skull, so when the rock-hard shiny surface of the radiotherapy table was clamped tightly up against it the result was waves of shooting pain. The agony was almost indescribable. I've had a baby with no pain relief and, believe me, that wasn't pleasant. But it was a different kind of pain – it was constructive pain, if you understand. When I was giving birth, I knew the reason for the pain and I also felt I could physically push it away as I pushed my baby out. But this was a magnitude of horror like I've never known. I began to sweat. Saliva flooded my mouth like a torrent. I was terrified I was going to vomit. Panic struck: how would I manage to vomit? I was clamped to the table and unable to even move my arms. The mask encompassed my shoulders and the tops of my arms.

The radiotherapist had explained that they could see me on camera. I could kick my legs and they'd stop the machine. But I was acutely aware that a) they were a few moments' sprint away should the worst happen and b) I needed this treatment done. I closed my eyes and tried to think of something to concentrate on. I recited my multiplication tables and tried to do the alphabet backwards.

The waves of hideous pain were joined by a burning feeling, akin to the one you get from new canvas trainers on hot feet, but it was on the inside of my head. The shafts of pain travelled, like dominoes falling, across the bones in my head in a clawing, ripping motion like one of those static-electricity balls with the fingers of shooting light. The large flying saucer moved on its enormous axis in slow motion. Each time it stopped the clunking noise was followed by the high-pitched sound I'd experienced before. But instead of the session lasting a matter of seconds this went on and on and on … The machine moved from my extreme left in a semicircle ending up on the right. I was dribbling out of both corners of my mouth (not attractive) and I knew I was making an animalistic noise that I hadn't realised I could produce.

What felt like a lifetime later, the noise ended and I could hear the radiotherapist's pounding feet as she ran to release me. As she unclipped the mask and I was able to lift my head away from the rock-like surface I knew I must look like a bug-eyed maniac.

'I can't stick that every day for six weeks,' I wailed. We agreed that I needed some strong pain relief, so I took my file and traipsed up the stairs to see the doctor. I made it to the top of the stairs before the retching began. I charged outside in time to vomit. Thankfully I didn't hit any unsuspecting patients and even managed to reach the bushes.

Staggering back into the heat of the hospital, I made it to the room where Dr Salib, one of the radiotherapy specialists, was waiting. He was kindly and sympathetic and wrote me a prescription for Solpadol. He instructed me to take them twenty minutes before the radiotherapy the following day.

Mercifully the pain had stopped as soon as the mask was removed, so I knew I wasn't going to be in constant pain.

The following day I presented myself feeling mildly smug. I'd downed my fizzy juice and was fully confident I wouldn't feel a thing.

Oh, how wrong was I?

Not only was the pain as bad, but the cancer was clearly not one bit happy about being zapped, so it was like a vicious and violent battle was taking place in my skull.

The painkillers hadn't helped at all. The shooting daggers were still there and the sense of panic was terrifying.

I grabbed my file once again and traipsed back up the stairs to see Dr Salib again. He explained that nerve pain could be difficult to banish and gave me some Difene to add to the Solpadol.

Joyously, I assumed the cocktail would solve the issue.

By the end of the week I was wiped out. Nothing seemed to even take the edge off the pain. I had a break over the weekend and arrived back in the hospital the following Monday filled with trepidation.

Professor Armstrong saw me. With his usual no-nonsense approach, he examined my head and neck and listened intently to my moaning and bleating.

He prescribed turbo-charged painkillers and pointed out that nothing was going to entirely relieve the pain until the tumour began to shrink. I spoke with the radiotherapists and they explained that they hoped to see some results by the end of the second week or the beginning of the third week. While it wasn't exactly what I wanted to hear, I was glad of the information.

An improvement wasn't set in stone by any stretch of the imagination, but it was a goal. The annoying part of all this was that I didn't need pain relief once I was finished on the radiotherapy table. So I was desperately trying to balance an optimal amount of relief without being out of my bin and unable to conduct myself in everyday life. I needed to be *compos mentis* enough to drive my car. (I never like anybody bringing me to or from my appointments. I feel if I go on my own, I'm more in control.) I also needed to be able to work.

I learned to time my painkillers, only taking them in the car on the journey into the hospital. That was a fabulous plan unless there was a delay with my appointment, which happened several times. As it's such a busy place, it's inevitable that times will alter. Some patients might need longer than anticipated, or indeed the machine can break down, meaning there'll be a backlog of patients. In those cases I had to sit, slightly pie-eyed, in the waiting room trying not to look as if I'd consumed a bottle of gin.

I brought my trusty laptop on all my visits. I'd sent my next novel, *The Summer Guest*, off to the publishers and they were busy getting it ready for a spring release. So I needed a new project. Something to keep my mind straight and give me a reason to focus.

I'd received so many letters from readers telling me how much they'd enjoyed my novel *Driving Home for Christmas* that I'd agreed to write a sequel. It would be my second novel for 2014, and it meant I could go to that special place where I was always happy – the land of tinsel, fairy lights, family dinners, baking and general frivolity. Once I started, it was like a light had been switched on inside my head again. I had an escape. I had an entire world that

I could immerse myself in while I either sat waiting or lay on the radiation table. Instead of concentrating on the pain and stress, I planned chapters or, in the case of the waiting room, I wrote those chapters. *The Heart of Winter* was the result of that time and it's a book that I'm both proud of and slightly bewildered by in equal measure! I'm bewildered as I can't quite believe I wrote an entire novel while I was being blasted. But hey, what else would I have done? Gone slowly insane perhaps? Yet again my publishers were astounding. By now my books were selling in the UK, so I had two editors. I still had Ciara but this time I had the wonderful guidance of Mari Evans across the water too. The book was due for release the following October, giving us plenty of time to plan and market it. I cannot express how cathartic my writing was for me at that time. I don't know how I would've managed without it. I cannot thank my publishers enough for backing me back then. To date, they've never turned me away or told me that they didn't want to look at my work. Quite the opposite – they embrace what I do and encourage me every step of the way. How lucky am I?

As the fractions continued so too did the pain. But I had my new focus and One Direction. The radiotherapists were incredibly kind to me – there's a CD player in the room with the machine and every day they'd put on One Direction at nightclub loudness so I could pretend I was at their concert. The mask was so tight I couldn't sing along, which is a good thing for all concerned, but I could wiggle my feet in time to the music and pretend I was dancing. I gritted my teeth and endured the pain, hoping with every fraction that the cancer was being killed.

Quite frankly, at that point one of us had to go. It was me or the cancer, and for the first time I wasn't certain whom it would be.

During the previous year I'd gotten to know a wonderfully fun and zany beauty writer by the name of Triona McCarthy. Triona is one of life's bubbly, beautiful beams of light. She sadly lost her younger sister Tricia to cancer and is very involved in fundraising for cancer charities. She told me about Breast Cancer Ireland and how they raise funds for cancer research. My ears pricked up. Over the years I've seen such amazing advances in medicine and I know

I am very lucky to benefit from them. Without modern medicine I wouldn't be here, end of.

Triona told me Breast Cancer Ireland were organising an event called Strictly against Breast Cancer. They hoped to sell one thousand tickets for a gala night planned for December. The idea was that Irish celebrities would pair up with and dance with breast cancer survivors in a *Strictly Come Dancing*-style show.

I signed up to dance. Don't ask me why, but I thought it would be a bit of diversion.

One of my bucket-list wishes has always been to perform that dance from *Dirty Dancing*. Patrick Swayze is a hero of mine and I, like most other women of a certain vintage, longed to be Baby and not left in the corner, even for a few minutes!

Rehearsals began in earnest. I honestly believed I could dance before that first lesson. Well, put it this way, I am the first onto the dance floor at a party or wedding and I adore it. But as the choreographers put us through our paces, I felt like my feet had been removed and instead I'd been left with two uncontrollably drunk creatures operating independently to my brain.

We were partnered up and given our dances. I was thrilled to be allowed do the end dance from *Dirty Dancing* and, along with Damian and our fabulous instructor Aideen, I got going.

At the best of times I'm fairly able bodied, but due to the radio-therapy my joints were as stiff as could be and I often felt like a clockwork dolly as I tried to master the moves.

Rehearsals officially took place twice a week, but Damian and I knew we needed to practise a little more so we'd have the routine off to a tee. He was incredibly patient with me, especially during the spins and lifts as waves of nausea washed over me.

The big lift, the one where I run and jump and he holds me over his head, was clearly what the audience would be waiting for. The very thought of it terrified and thrilled us in equal measure. The instruction was that I was to run and jump, and Damian was to catch me at either side of my hips and hoist me into the air, bless him.

In the beginning it all seemed like an impossible feat. I was like a sack of wet sand with as much spring in my step as a whale. But slowly we got better and I rose higher. Thinking we'd have one last solo session at the dance studio, we booked a slot and turned up, vowing to nail it for once and for all. There were only ten days till show time.

As I ran across the studio and jumped and dove over his head there was a loud crack. Damian held me aloft and I almost flew directly over his back in glee.

He put me down and grasped his hand.

'What?' I asked in alarm.

'Ah, nothing, it'll be fine,' he assured me.

We went our separate ways, me to my radiotherapy and to work and Damian back to his office – or so I thought. That evening he texted me a photo of his hand in plaster! He'd broken his thumb – or, more specifically, I had broken Damien.

We soldiered on but it was decided we couldn't do the famous lift. Instead we did a run-and-jump-and-twirl-around sort of effort. Not quite as dramatic but it was enough to keep the audience mildly amused.

On the day of the show we pitched up at Dublin's Convention Centre for a dress rehearsal. I knew from the moment I woke that I was harbouring an infection. My chest was rattling and I knew I was on borrowed time before the chills started and I'd end up either in hospital or in bed at home. I got through the practice run and Aisling and Sam from Breast Cancer Ireland had kindly booked me a room in a nearby hotel to lie down. I excused myself, saying I was having a little rest, and dashed to the hospital where they dosed me with antibiotics and painkillers. The show must go on!

The hair stylists and the crew from Makeup Forever had some job on their hands that night, but they did wonderful work and I looked a hell of a lot better than I felt! The atmosphere in the room when we ran onto the stage was simply electric. They say we should all do things that scare us, as it's character building. This was terrifying and exhilarating in equal measure. I can honestly say, hand on heart, that it was one of the most amazing experiences of my life. A shed-load of money was raised for cancer research and Damian and I were thrilled to take third place! That glass trophy takes pride of place on the shelf in my office. It was tough physically, but that night and the build-up most certainly helped me through a very dark time.

Mercifully, as the fractions were drawing to an end, the tumour on my head began to shrink. Once the shrinkage started the process was miraculous. Day by day I could feel the hard, marbled mass melting. The nodes in my neck were mostly gone and, although my skin was pink and fried looking, the light was beginning to shine through from the end of the tunnel.

I was exhausted both mentally and physically. The pain in my head had eased a little. The scale of ouch had reduced from sledge-hammer level to red-hot-needles-in-the-skull level, which was more bearable in the greater scheme of things.

Christmas was a welcome interval that thankfully stopped the radiation fractions for a while. I was cooked on one side and knew I had to go back for the other side to be done. But it was a relief to have a break. The trooping in and out of the hospital every day had worn thin. I was using astronomical amounts of petrol – a First-World problem, I know, but all the same it was noticeable. The extra financial drains add up pretty swiftly and even paying for the car park each day was a hassle. Thankfully the hospital I attend for radiation has now introduced a system whereby patients can buy a laminated car-parking ticket. This enables them to park without having to root for change each day.

For the first time during my cancer story I had a Christmas where cancer tried to overshadow proceedings. I tried not to let it get to me. We still celebrated royally. I still put up four trees around the house, and I made sure we had as much fun as humanly possible.

Yet again we all headed off for our now traditional New Year's Eve break at Dromoland Castle. I crawled in the door wearied and left four days later feeling rejuvenated.

But I was burnt on one side of my neck and my head was aching. I was also half-bald. Yes, you've read it right. It is possible to be semi-bald. I hadn't realised that radiation could cause alopecia, but guess what? It can and does, and needless to say it happened to me. It stands to reason that frying the back of one's head is going to deftly kill the hair as it stamps on the cancer. So I looked the way I always did from the front, but if so much as a gust of wind appeared, my thinning hair would lift to reveal my shiny, bald head at the back! It was easily rectified with a strip of clip-in hair that attached to what I had left. No big deal in the greater scheme of things. I was simply astonished to realise that radiation could make me bald after I'd gone to such lengths to hold on to my hair during the previous chemotherapy!

Professor Armstrong ordered fresh scans and we were both over-joyed to see the results. The radiotherapy had worked like a dream. Even better, I didn't have any problems with my salivary gland and my skin was healing nicely. I was and still am incredibly grateful that I had such an astute and precise doctor looking after me.

By 5 February I was back in my mask on the radiotherapy table. This time, praise the Lord, there was no pain involved. All the tumours from the back of my head had been eradicated so I was only being zapped on the length of my neck and into my collarbone. I presume it was due to the previous build-up of radiotherapy but this second bout hit me like a sledgehammer from the word go. It was as if my body recognised the treatment and jumped directly into action with making me feel dreadful.

The darkness that hovers over many of us in life could possibly have descended upon me at that moment. For the first time ever I could appreciate what it might feel like to be depressed.

I've said it before and I'll say it again now. There is someone watching over me. Every time I've felt as if I could hit rock bottom, something happened and the rainbows appeared once more, colouring my world with splashes of positivity.

This period was no different. The week before I finished treatment, just as I was beginning to feel as if I ought to be crawling on my hands and knees in a fug of cancer-induced misery, I got a call from Jessie Collins, the editor of *Irish Tatler* magazine at that time. She wanted to interview me and put me on the front cover!

When I answered my mobile phone, I was sitting outside the radiotherapy-cum-torture chamber with my laptop balanced on my knees, writing. I don't mind admitting, I grinned like a goon.

'Can your photographer Photoshop my neck?' I asked. 'It looks like it's been boiled in oil.' Jessie assured me that wouldn't be an issue. Barry McCall was taking the shots so I knew I was in expert hands. If you don't know Barry, take it from me: he is a magician with a camera and could make a bulldog look beautiful.

The day of the photo shoot, I was due in hospital at 5.30 p.m., so I had enough time beforehand to go to the Shelbourne Hotel in Dublin. This salubrious hotel is nestled at the edge of St Stephen's Green and has hosted many rich and famous souls over the years. Right at the top of this majestic building is the most sublime suite imaginable. Jessie had set up an entire village of people to complete the shoot. Christine Lucignano from Chanel did my face. When I say this lady is a make-up artist it doesn't describe what she actually does. She's a wizard with a brush! Dylan Bradshaw was in charge of the tiny amount of hair I owned. He asked me what kind of look I wanted and my only wish was that I didn't look mumsy. Nobody wants to be on the cover of a magazine looking frumpy, let's face it.

'The camera will be pointed at your face. So nobody will know you've no hair at the back,' he said logically. So he backcombed it and teased it up in a funky eighties-meets-party-girl style.

Aisling Farinella was in charge of styling so she had a rail of clothes that had been crafted by the gods. Green leather trousers, tulip-shaped skirts and a breathtaking ball gown made from Aztec fabric. All were by couture designers and were showstopper pieces. Folks, I'd have died happy if the good Lord had taken me at that moment.

I fell in love with the moss-green leather jeans and if I'd had the money I would've bought them. I still think about them longingly all these years later. Someday I will have the cash to spend on green leather – I live in hope!

I've known Barry McCall for a long time. In fact, I met him on holiday in the Canary Islands when we were eighteen. Neither of us would've guessed we'd meet in such stunning surroundings twenty-odd years later. I can assure you, the Shelbourne was a damn sight nicer than the apartments we were in all those years ago! It was wonderful to have a photographer I felt comfortable with. Every time I allowed myself to think that I was having my picture taken for the cover of a glossy magazine I had an out-of-body experience. It was utterly surreal (in a good way). The whole experience was just like being a princess for the day. The interview followed and I then drove to St Vincent's with my funky hair, a full face of make-up and my own clothes back on. The last fraction of treatment that day was a true celebration in so many ways.

My life had been taken over by radiotherapy treatments. I had struggled to fit work, family, friends and general existing into the week. Cancer can be damn time-consuming, you know.

The following week, the sense of freedom without the daily hospital appointments was wonderful and I felt like a teenager at the beginning of the summer holidays. I suddenly had all this time to spare!

A month later I went back to the Blackrock Clinic to see my oncologist, David Fennelly. We were at a crossroads. All the lumps and bumps were gone bar one tiny one in my neck. Professor Armstrong was of the opinion that it would go on its own. It had been royally zapped so there was no logic to it still being viable.

I was offered a choice. Either I could go away and see what happened next with regular monitoring or I could go back on Avastin chemotherapy.

After a logical and open conversation with David, I decided I would prefer the safety net of Avastin. The side effects weren't debilitating and I had always tolerated the drug well in the past. I didn't want to dodge the treatment and end up regretting it bitterly a year down the road.

We agreed I would start back on three-weekly infusions. By this point it was May of 2014. I was back in my home away from home, aka Blackrock Clinic Oncology day unit. I was freshly aware of the family atmosphere and the warmth of the staff. I have never minded going in there and count myself incredibly lucky that I have such caring people at my back.

Three days after that first infusion of Avastin, the final rogue lump on my neck disappeared. I was over the moon and felt we had made the right call to administer the drug again.

In August of that year, Cian came home one evening and stood inside the front door, calling out to us. We all appeared, peeking either out of the kitchen or down the stairs. There, in his arms, was a tiny, blond, curly ball of fuzz.

'It's a golden doodle puppy,' he said with a grin.

Needless to say Sacha and Kim were magnetised to him instantly.

Once we put him down on the kitchen floor and showed him the cardigan that Cian had been given from the breeder that the mummy dog had slept on with him he seemed quite happy.

His name changed a thousand times over that first week. Eventually we agreed on Herbie. Tom the cat didn't seem too phased by him and they became friends quite quickly. I've never been a dog person. I always preferred cats and didn't quite get the doggy fascination – until I met Herbie! He has stolen all our hearts and is the most cheerful, loving and astonishingly responsive creature imaginable. The pleasure he derives from a walk is contagious. He cost us a fortune in the beginning. He ate his way through a couple of hundred euros worth of shoes, UGG boots and even a kitchen windowsill. But he's worth it!

Chapter 44

That's Life!

My writing career was hurtling along nicely. My novel *Perfect Wives* and then the second Christmas one, *The Heart of Winter*, hit the shelves in Ireland, the UK, Australia and New Zealand. I continued to appear on TV and radio and was enjoying every minute of it.

Sacha and Kim were into their teens and life was moving onward and upwards for us all. Cian's business, his triathlon emporium Base2Race, survived the recession and we were both in jobs we enjoyed.

My work with Breast Cancer Ireland continued, and in 2014 I was a judge for another Strictly against Breast Cancer, which was far easier than dancing! I was privileged to be invited to the research lab where the scientists were making massive strides in cancer treatments. There I met with an astonishing group of young, bright innovators who explained how the money was being spent. Not only did I learn a whole host of things about how cancer treatments were changing, but also they were able to tell me that it was highly unlikely that my cancer would ever spread to my organs.

Apparently cancer cells, when they travel around the body, either have the strength and ability to permeate organs or they don't. As research continues, they are slowly beginning to be able to identify which ones are 'organ invaders'. They said my history would lead them to believe that my type of breast cancer cannot invade my organs. Obviously I would need proper tests to confirm this, but it made total sense to me. I sincerely hope they're right.

As an ambassador for Breast Cancer Ireland I try to get involved in as many initiatives as possible to raise money for research. In line with that, I agreed to take part in their Feel Yourselfie campaign. This involved a photo shoot with the wonderful Barry McCall once more. I pitched up with a gang of celebs and we promptly took our tops off and covered our modesty with our own hands. It was all very tastefully done and we were happy that it would send out the right message. The photographs appeared in the *Sunday Independent* magazine.

The night after the photo shoot I called my lovely friend, TV3's *Ireland AM* anchor Sinéad Desmond, in a vaguely numbed stupor.

'What did we do today?' I asked. Sinéad giggled and said she was glad I felt mildly traumatised too. It's not that easy to take one's clothes off and have a photo taken! Still, it helped raise much-needed funds for cancer research, so that was the whole point. To say my teenagers were not impressed when the paper came out that Sunday is putting it mildly. As any parent of a teenaged son or daughter will tell you, we are a constant source of embarrassment, so appearing semi-nude in the paper was probably a heinous crime against street cred!

By October 2015 my body was showing signs that had become all too familiar. This time I had pain in my right shoulder as well. As the months passed, a huge tumour the size of an egg formed on the left side of my neck. More appeared on the back of my head, the right side of my neck, under my right arm and at the front of my collarbone. David Fennelly told me about a new drug he had heard of called Veliparib, which is a PARP inhibitor.

PARP inhibitors are the new way forward for cancer patients. The way they work is pretty complex and quite honestly I don't understand it fully. But my basic and blonde explanation of what they do is this: when cancer forms in the body, the immune system rushes in to see if there's something that needs fixing. Cancer is a nasty and horrible creature so it tells the immune system to go away – nothing to see here, move along, thank you. So the immune system leaves it and the cancer is allowed to grow and spread. What a PARP inhibitor does is act as a buffer between the cancer and the immune system. It's the good cop, and it says to the immune system, 'Wait! Don't listen to the cancer, there is something here and you need to tackle it.' So PARP inhibitors are wonderful and innovative things that could change the face of cancer treatment. Instead of going in and obliterating the cancer the way chemotherapy and radiation do, these treatments could help cancer patients to fix their own bodies. Magical, right?

So I waited and waited and waited while my team tried to source Veliparib. Essentially, this drug was designed for patients with triple negative breast cancer brought on by the BRCA1 gene. That's me, in a nutshell. I tick all those boxes! I was so excited and the best part was that they were tablets. No IV drips and I could take them at home with minimal hospital visits. The other wonderful aspect was that I could potentially be on this drug indefinitely, as it could possibly stop the cancer from returning.

I couldn't wait for the tablets to arrive.

Meanwhile, as the weeks turned to months, the cancer grew and grew like an untamed weed inside my body. The pain in my neck and shoulder became paralysing. I was taking nerve-blocker painkillers mixed with Solpadeine and was pretty much bed bound. I was swollen to the point that I no longer had a collarbone and I honestly didn't recognise the person staring back at me in the mirror. My weight went to a new high. I hadn't been this heavy since I was pregnant, yet I wasn't eating anything different at all.

Just as I feared I might spiral beneath the floor into a big black hole of anxiety, Sherise Hobbs, my London editor, rang to let me know that I'd been nominated for a RONA award. These prestigious awards are held in London and were to be presented by author and TV personality Fern Britton. Knowing I was on the edge and not able for much due to the hideous pain I was in, I debated whether or not I'd manage a trip to London. But I knew if I didn't go I'd always regret it. So, pumped to the eyeballs with nerve blockers, I ventured to London on 7 March. I had just learned my novel *The Perfect Gift* was number one in the charts, so I was already on a high.

Sherise Hobbs, my agent Sheila Crowley and I arrived at the stunning Gladstone Library in Whitehall Place. I was surrounded by authors and the glitterati of the literature world – should they be called the literati?

After a champagne reception we took to our table and waited for the awards to be announced. I was up for Epic Novel of the Year. I assumed I hadn't a chance in hell of winning. I was overwhelmed by the talent in the room and was literally grateful to have been let in the door at all.

When Fern Britton called my name and said that *The Secrets We Share* had won, I was rooted to the spot. Sheila and Sherise had to nudge me and almost tip me out of my chair to go to the stage to accept my award. Apparently I made a speech. I don't remember if it was coherent or not, I was so dumbfounded! I still find it incredible that I won – the beautiful crystal star award is twinkling at me from a shelf in my office right now.

The Perfect Gift continued to dominate the number-one spot in Ireland and I was so grateful to my writing world for making me see that, no matter how bad things were with my health, there was still a light in my life.

The happiness was dimmed a couple of weeks later, however.

On 24 March 2016 my beloved aunt Mitzi died of leukaemia. She was the nearest in age to Mum and I had spent much of my childhood in her house. Her eldest son, my cousin Fionn, and I are only a few months apart in age and we shared so many wonderful memories growing up. Mitzi was doing brilliantly – or so we'd all thought. She'd had a bone-marrow transplant and everything was going well. She seemed to be getting better and then all of a sudden we were told she had two weeks to live. I landed from London after the RONAs and brought my award to show her. I was shocked by her appearance. She was jaundiced and sunken and I knew there and then that she was on the way out.

Mum was utterly shattered. They were kindred spirits – they went to ceramics classes together and shared a love of art. They weren't just sisters: they were friends. Our entire extended family was united in grief as we spent as much time with Mitzi as we could. We took it in turns to sit with her either at home (if she managed to get back there for a couple of hours in the afternoon) or in the hospice. Right up until the last moment, she maintained her quirky sense of humour and was still cracking jokes until the night before she passed away. During our final conversation at the hospice, I leaned over to kiss her as she lay wasting away in front of our very eyes. As I said goodbye, she held my hand and told me, with a cheeky smile, that I was to continue to wear bright-pink lipstick.

'Never stop being a pink girl,' she said. My tears turned to laughter as I nodded and smiled back.

Her bravery and acceptance of what lay ahead for her was astonishing. I miss her every day and I hope she has met with Neil and Helen and her baby son whom she lost to a cot death. She told us all he was waiting for her and that he had beckoned to her several days before she died. I hope he was there to meet her and that he's minding her now.

Once again I was ravaged by survivor's guilt. All the thoughts I'd had when Neil died returned with vigor. Why had she been taken while I was still here? It didn't seem fair and it didn't make much sense. I could have wallowed in that dark thought indefinitely, but I knew that I had to stop thinking that way. I have always been uber aware of the fact that I am incredibly lucky to be alive, that I am blessed to have survived – nobody recognises that more clearly than me. If I'm going to throw that away and allow sadness and guilt to take over, I might as well go out into the back garden and dig a hole. I feel as if it's my duty to keep going and embrace the time I've been given with my family and loved ones.

Eventually, in May 2016, the magic tablets I'd been waiting for arrived. I was to take four twice a day. They promised to be kinder to my system than chemotherapy and work even more deftly. The doctors and nurses were so excited and I couldn't wait to get going. I felt it couldn't go wrong.

The first dose I took hit me like a smack in the face. I can tell you the exact second the drug hit my system. I'd left the hospital and was in the supermarket doing my grocery shopping when, all of a sudden, I was very thankful for the handle of the trolley. The shop began to spin as the sounds of the busy supermarket droned in and out. All I can equate it to was being blind drunk on tequila as a teenager. But this time it happened in the flick of a switch.

Somehow I managed to stagger to the cash desk, pay for the food and make it to the car. Knowing I should probably call someone to come and get me, I did what all stubborn people do, and I drove home very slowly with one eye shut and the windows open. Even though I was at a slow, crawling pace, looking back, I know I was lucky to make it home in one piece. The teenagers were in school but Herbie and Tom were there to greet me. We sat on the sofa and, as my world continued to spin at an ever-increasing pace, the furries were thrilled to have somebody to snuggle with and seemed oblivious to my distress.

I hoped the initial effect would ease and that I'd get used to the drug. But as the doses accumulated in my system, things went from bad to worse. Two days later I was vomiting uncontrollably with crippling vertigo and the worst headache I have ever experienced. My brain felt as if it were trying to escape my head, possibly through both ears.

I phoned my oncologist and he agreed I should drop the dose from four tablets to three.

That night as I tipped the tablets into my hand (they were luminous green with menacing black stripes) I felt like crying. I was so terrified of taking them that I feared for my life. My hands shook as I raised them to my mouth and I literally had to stop myself from gagging as I swallowed.

I was so sick and in so much pain that I honestly thought about flushing them down the toilet – every single one – and pretending I'd taken them.

The only thing that kept me going at that time was the thought that they must be doing amazing things with the cancer. If the effects were so dramatic on my body, surely the cancer was having an even worse time – right?

Sadly, three tablets weren't a whole heap better than four. I still couldn't move or get out of bed. I was so dizzy and sick with a thumping headache that I couldn't actually function. So I was allowed to drop the dose to two, twice a day.

While the sickness abated somewhat, I was faced with a whole new problem – an insatiable need to eat large amounts. If I didn't eat a substantial meal before taking the tablets, I'd be as sick as a dog. The nausea only let up when I ate. It's usually the opposite with other drugs such as chemotherapy – with that, eating large amounts would be detrimental and would certainly cause more vomiting. But not with this drug. The more food I consumed, the more normal I felt. So I found myself stuffing double portions into my tummy. In ordinary circumstances I have a healthy appetite. I have never eaten like a bird, nor am I one of those people who can survive on tiny amounts of food. But this new form of binging was on a massive scale. Unsurprisingly, as a result I was bloated and felt similarly to when I was about six or seven months pregnant. Unsurprisingly, my body ballooned as I piled on weight. Any time I tried to curb my food intake I began to feel sick and constant vomiting ensued. Ooh, what a fabulous choice! I could opt for being either twice my usual size or violently sick.

I battled on with the tablets for eight weeks. I had regular blood tests and they revealed that my cells were all within normal range. So I wasn't neutropenic or lacking in platelets. That was fantastic, but there was one hitch. The lumps and tumours weren't reducing in size. The pain wasn't going and I was still feeling toxic. I couldn't keep up with eating huge amounts of food, so in turn I was battling vicious headaches and fighting constant nausea.

David Fennelly issued new scans and they revealed what we'd all suspected – Veliparib wasn't doing what it ought. In fact it wasn't working at all. The cancer was literally giving us two fingers on the scan. It was laughing in our faces and growing and spreading like wildfire.

I felt defeated and utterly deflated (in reality I was very much inflated, but you know what I mean). The magic cure wasn't so magic after all. By now, the pain had halted every part of my life. My right shoulder was so swollen that my collarbone was no longer visible. The tumours were huge on both sides of my neck, but the one on the left-hand side was scary. It bulged to the size of a kiwi fruit and looked like a hiding alien. Another golf-ball-sized nasty had popped up at the front of my neck, low down near the throat where there is normally a crevice. It was rock hard and growing by the day.

I had shooting pains down my right arm and from my right shoulder up into my head. Another massive Henry was flourishing on the right at the back of my skull. That nasty bastard was sending nice electric-shock-style shots of pain down the back of my neck.

I like to think I have a fairly decent pain threshold. After all, I managed to have a baby with zero pain relief, not to mention getting through the hideous radiation. But I was back in nerve-pain hell. This time it was so severe it made me want to croon on the floor like a wounded animal. Aoibheann, Sinéad and Dr Rachel at the Oncology day unit were sympathetic and lovely and provided me with a whole range of painkillers. I worked my way up the scale until I was sandwiching Solpadeine with Lyrica nerve blockers. They worked wonderfully for a while until the pain rose above them. The dose was raised three times and yet I still couldn't function.

Pain is one thing, but it was devastating to know that the cancer was progressing. I could see the tumours getting bigger, harder and more aggressive with each passing day. I couldn't lie on either side at night and was forced to prop myself up awkwardly with pillows. I took sleeping pills hoping they would knock me out for a few hours. While they offered a little respite, the pain continuously woke me.

While taking the Veliparib, I had literally lain like a wooden dolly counting the days until the treatment worked. When the scans confirmed that it wasn't working I was floored.

This had a profound effect on my children. For the first time ever, I couldn't hide the seriousness of the cancer. I couldn't jolly them along and act as if it was OK. The cancer was taking over and I felt as if it was winning.

Dr Fennelly took the decision to put me onto chemotherapy immediately. At that time I would've agreed to pretty much anything. So in July 2016 I began a course of Cisplatin and Avastin. As Cisplatin can cause kidney damage, I had to go to the hospital for a sleepover in order to have fluids for eight hours before treatment started.

When I checked into hospital for the first round of chemotherapy I was like a small child at Christmas. I could tell that the medical team were a little baffled by my excitement. I was grinning from ear to ear and couldn't wait to start. Why? Because it had worked in the past, so I was pinning my hopes on its getting rid of this blasted cancer. Although it's no friend of mine, I know chemotherapy's track record. No matter how awful it made me feel, it always killed the cancer. I'd suffered so much sickness and pain in the previous few months that I figured nothing could be as bad.

I was right – to a point ...

Within two treatments, which were given routinely every two weeks via a drip, the tumours started to recede, taking the unbearable pain with them. I cannot begin to explain how satisfying it is to literally see the tumours melt away under my skin.

It's a blessing in one way and a curse in another that my cancer is actually visible. When it's growing and flourishing and having a happy time taking over my body, it's terrifying to see how swiftly it can multiply. But when the correct treatment takes hold and starts to obliterate it and I can feel the cancer disappearing, there's no better sensation.

As the chemotherapy treatments progressed, there was a cumulative effect. The nausea and life-stopping tiredness built week by week. In turn my bloods began to show signs of weakness. And another strange thing was beginning to happen. My hearing was muffled for a few days after each treatment.

I reported this to the nurses and was promptly sent off to visit Ms Aoife Walsh, the audiologist. Together with her assistant Nuala, they put my ears through their paces. I was put into a soundproof booth on a red chair (thankfully not one that tips backwards like Graham Norton's). I felt a bit like a contestant on *Mr & Mrs*, as I had earphones placed on.

'Press this each time you hear a noise,' Nuala said as she handed me a little buzzer.

The noises ranged from high pitched to low and dull.

Thankfully I passed the test with flying colours and Aoife confirmed that my ears were doing well. Apparently Cisplatin chemotherapy can damage the tiny hairs on the inside of the ears, causing hearing loss. So although I was experiencing some muffled sensations for a couple of days after my treatment, my ears were holding up.

Chemotherapy has a cumulative effect, and although the tumours were disappearing one by one, which was totally amazing, my body was beginning to feel it, big time, as the chemotherapy built up in my system.

By treatment number six, I knew I was headed for trouble. I was losing my hair bit by bit – each time I brushed it, more fell out. If I allowed the shower water to hit my scalp, I'd shed an entire layer of hair so it looked like a blond spider was attempting to squash itself down the plughole. I spent my time picking my hair off clothing and furniture and spitting out strands of it. Why is it that hair likes to jump into my mouth? It's completely gross but it must be something to do with lips being moist … Ugh!

Hair loss is a First-World problem in the greater scheme of things and, believe me, it wasn't exactly my most pressing issue. So I knew I'd have to grin and bear it. I replenished my supply of clip-in hairpieces and I became particularly attached to a wide plait that could be worn like an Alice band. This was a marvellous invention, as it covered a large amount of baldness on the sides and top of my head. It was soft and light and perfect for accompanying my little twisted bun hairpiece, which I secured at the nape of my neck. I also became a slave to Batiste Dry Shampoo with a hint of colour. Yes, it comes in brilliant blond and it really and truly works. Not only did it freshen my diminishing hair, but it added a bit of brightness so my scalp wasn't totally shiny and glaringly obvious. It plumps up the hair too, so even the thinnest scraping of hair can look quite acceptable. This marvellous stuff comes in several shades. I don't have personal experience of the brunette version but the blond one is second to none.

Knowing that my poor fronds were shedding and disappearing down the plughole with every wash, I applied some lateral thinking and I stopped washing it. I know that sounds utterly disgusting, but when you've only got a spattering of candy floss-like hair, it honestly doesn't need much interference. I hasten to add that I still showered once and sometimes twice a day, so I wasn't pongy, I promise. I crossed my fingers and toes that I'd hold on to enough hair to make it through the chemotherapy cycle without having to resort to a full-blown wig. I'd worn them before and was glad of them, but when there's a chance of being able to make do, it seems like a better option. Perhaps it was psychological too – if I held on to some of my hair, I wasn't being totally stamped on by the chemotherapy …

That was a silly notion, really, because it was becoming starkly obvious to me and the medical team that the chemotherapy was indeed getting the better of me. If we were running in a race against one another, the chemotherapy was at the finish line, full of energy, blowing raspberries at me as I plodded exhaustedly from the starting point.

Knowing I was beginning to fade, my medical team asked me to attend the hospital for mid-cycle bloods. So a week after my sixth treatment I did just that. As they'd suspected, things weren't great. I was neutropenic with a grand total of zero white blood cells. My magnesium levels were dangerously low and I was lacking platelets too. No wonder I was so wrecked.

So it was decided that I needed to stay in overnight and have several bags of goodies to build me back up again. Normally I am very naughty when it comes to spending time in hospital. I'll do everything in my power to escape and get home. But I was so tired and sick that I reckon I would've agreed to go to prison at that point. I packed my bag and drove to the hospital. Normally I stay in my clothes until bedtime, stubbornly refusing to look like a patient. Yes, I know it's ridiculous but it's a game I like to play. This time I was straight into my pyjamas and into bed. I was ready to do what they wanted me to, just so long as I could feel a bit more human.

It had been a long time since I'd had a blood transfusion, but I had a vague recollection of feeling marvellous afterwards, of being filled with energy and ready to kick ass once more. So I signed the consent forms and was quite excited to think that I might feel better soon.

As the blood seeped into my port, I had a little fiction-writer's moment. I sat in a mild stupor wondering who might have donated the first and then second bag of blood I was receiving. Was it a young man who was full of energy? Was it a college student or a lawyer? Was it a farmer or a nun? After a few moments of pondering I settled on feeling enormously grateful to whoever it was. I marvelled at the fact that someone I didn't know had taken the time to go and donate their nutritious and healthy blood so that someone ill like me could get better. It's hard to fathom unless you've been the recipient of a blood transfusion, but it's hugely humbling and made me want to shout 'thank you' from the roof of the hospital.

I've mentioned before that I'm not a crier – I rarely well up – but as I sat and watched the bags of blood drip into my body, I sobbed. It's impossible for me to portray how grateful I felt. Receiving a blood transfusion is all down to human kindness. It happens because totally selfless individuals make a point of helping others. I found that quite overwhelming. I really wished the process wasn't anonymous. I still want to thank the person or people who helped me that day. I wish I could bake them a tray of brownies and write them a card. I hope blood donors know what amazing people they really are.

Once the two blood transfusions were drip-fed into me, it was time for a large bag of magnesium. The nurses had been concerned that I might feel ill during or after the blood transfusion. They repeatedly took my blood pressure and checked that I wasn't feeling shaky or sick. They checked my temperature and made sure I wasn't going to collapse in a heap on the floor. But nobody expected the magnesium to cause any hassle.

Of course, that's exactly what it did. Can I do anything normally? No, is the short answer. About an hour into the three-hour infusion I began to feel the effects.

I was as sick as a dog: my stomach was like a washing machine with cramps that doubled me over. Then came the headaches. Oh dear Lord, I honestly thought my brain was slowly inflating and readying itself to explode inside my throbbing skull. The painful thudding went on all night, along with flushing skin, as the washing-machine tummy kept going only to be joined by a few leg cramps for a bit of extra excitement. I asked for paracetamol, which provided as much relief as a Jelly Tot. So I had to sit it out for four hours until I was safely allowed to have more paracetamol, this time in the form of Solpadeine. Mercifully, by close to midnight, I was given two of those magic fizzy tablets dissolved in water. The bitter, bubbly taste was never so welcome. I wouldn't have been as happy if they'd handed me a glass of vintage Bollinger.

By that point I could feel my eyeballs rolling in their sockets, such was the pain in my head. I managed a bit of sleep, but I know I was making involuntary groaning/moaning noises that didn't sound exactly human. Thankfully I was in a private room and didn't have to inflict my pitiful suffering on anyone else. I was mortified for myself, which is really a bad state of affairs. Diarrhoea joined the party and I spent the night dragging the drip in and out of the bathroom. Retching uncontrollably followed, meaning I was flushed in the face with bloodshot eyes and therefore looking as if I'd been beaten up. Not my finest hour. Suffice it to say, I'm not a fan of magnesium and believe it should only be used intravenously to torture nasty people.

I escaped from hospital the following lunchtime and scurried home, driving with one eye shut. Yes, I probably should have accepted one of the many offers of a lift, but my car was there and I wanted to get home without delay. Also, and probably most importantly, I'm incredibly stubborn and wasn't going to give in!

The following day, I ran away to Connemara with Mum and Herbie the dog. The teenagers had pressing engagements with friends and Cian was working so they didn't join us. I am bad at leaving my kids to their own devices and always imagine that some great tragedy will befall both of them if I'm not around. But the reality is that they predominantly crave the company of their friends and only need me for money, lifts to places that aren't on the bus or train route and sporadic sympathy if something goes wrong. Cian was available to dash from work if there was a fallout and I gave them enough money to avoid starvation, but not enough to allow ruination, while making them aware I was available on the other end of the phone.

Mum and I chatted non-stop, while pulling over for regular refreshments so Herbie could cock his leg and have a drink of water. The journey took hours longer than usual but we arrived feeling stress free, armed with ready meals for dinner. Knowing we wouldn't see another soul for the evening, we got into our pyjamas and sat in deckchairs with our books, inhaling the deliciously clear, salty air and marvelling at the view of the rocky bay opposite the house.

Connemara is one of those rare locations that has pockets of totally unspoiled areas. Our cottage is perched on an incline with rolling hills of green mottled land to the rear and a clear view of a tiny bay to the front. A short stone pier stretches lazily into the water as dark spinach-coloured seaweed hugs the large boulders that sit at random like sleeping giants around a pebble-filled beach. Unless the weather is particularly wild (which is also astonishing to watch), the water looks like glass. Seagulls frequent the area, creating a fabulous natural spectacle as they dive for fish suppers.

The sounds couldn't be better if they were dubbed in through Bose speakers! There are cows mooing in the distance with sheep bleating woolly answers and the intermittent baying of donkeys. It probably sounds as if I'm making that up, but I swear that's what we hear as we sit outside our cottage! That and the sound of silence – it's blissful and oh-so-good for the soul.

Herbie is terrified of sheep, something we discovered as he came eyeball to eyeball with one on his first ever visit. The sheep bleated at him through the makeshift fence from the field next door and he literally nearly lost his reason. He reversed at a thousand miles an hour and ran, stricken, to hide behind my leg! So now he stays well back from his woolly cousins and plays with Luther, the waggy-tailed black Labrador belonging to Steven and Loretta who owned the house before us.

A night's sleep in this kind of tranquillity is like five nights of good sleep back home all rolled into one. So I always seem to wake feeling a little lighter than before.

The next morning, after a breakfast of duck eggs from the farm up the road, we set out for our walk on the beach.

There are lots of beaches in the area but our favourite is Gurteen Bay. With smooth golden sand, this place could be the Caribbean when the sun shines. If we humans like it at Gurteen, it's only the tip of the iceberg compared to how Herbie feels. The second we pitch up there he starts to get excited. After letting him out of the car, he inevitably shoots off and gallops around in a wide circle before doing ecstatic roly-polys on the sand. He literally makes us laugh out loud as he snuffles in piles of mermaid's purse in blissful delight. There's nothing quite like seeing the smiling, goony glee of a dog! The fresh sea air and the clear vistas of the Ten Ben mountain ranges and miles of ocean are the best therapy I know.

That day as we were walking out along the beach the sun was shining. I knew my energy levels weren't great, so I was totally out of breath after a few steps. The frustration from wanting to walk but finding it really difficult to keep going hit me hard. I literally wanted to stamp my feet and shout obscenities … Not that I had the energy for that either! I resisted and instead chose to walk for a bit, stop for a bit, walk for a bit and stop again – annoying, but better than sitting down all day.

I returned in plenty of time for the next and penultimate chemotherapy session. Figuring I would be in tip-top shape after the blood transfusions and the nasty bag of magnesium, I was floored when the nurses said I was still in a bad way. In spite of the transfusions and infusions I was back to square one. I was still neutropenic, my magnesium levels were in the doldrums again and I was lacking platelets. So chemotherapy had to be held off. I wanted to lie on the floor and have a tantrum and shout at St David that he was to administer the chemotherapy no matter what. That I would take the hit … That I would stay in bed for two weeks until the next one, if that was required. I would've sold my soul to the devil to get that bag of chemotherapy over and done with. But I knew having a meltdown wouldn't do any good. It was too dangerous to treat me, so instead I found myself hooked up to another large bag of magnesium. I felt like the naughtiest girl in the school who was being punished for putting dog poo in the headmaster's shoes!

The magnesium was now public enemy number one – my greatest hate, taking over from radiation to the back of the head. I tried to pretend it wasn't there. I tried to tell my head that it was only a bag of fluids, so there was no need to become all achy. I warned my tummy that it wasn't to get all washing machine-y and sick. But it soon became obvious that it wasn't a mind-over-matter thing. An hour later I was in the horrors once more. My skin seemed like it was on fire, my head felt like it was separating and the hideous dull thumping had returned. My eyes were swollen underneath and I honestly thought I was going to slither off my chair and onto the floor into a dark, oozing puddle of misery. I got some pain relief for my head, but nothing seemed to work for the stomach cramps and subsequent dashing to the bathroom. I did my best to look like I was fine and it worked – reluctantly, the nurses allowed me to drive home. They did suggest a sleepover, but I couldn't bear the thought of another night in a crunchy hospital bed with a drip attached to me.

So I crawled home in the car, with the promise of a soft, soothing pillow and my own bed leading me on. I went straight in the front door and directly under the duvet. If I were in a Monopoly game I wouldn't have passed Go and I wouldn't have collected two hundred euros. It was a swift and dogged action that involved peeling off my jeans and socks and sinking into bed with a happy sigh. I couldn't and didn't move (bar several swift exits to the bathroom) for twenty-four hours. I had a horrible taste in my mouth, no energy and I felt as weak as a kitten. My old pal Solpadeine had to be called upon once more and I know two things as a result of that experience. Firstly, magnesium is an evil bastard. Secondly, Solpadeine is my best friend. I would give it my last fiver and drive a thousand miles to get it.

Sacha and Kim were amazing during those awful hours. Sacha, who towers over me and is stocky in build, still climbs into bed beside me for chats. He hugs me freely and makes me laugh out loud each and every day. He brings me coffee, tea, water or what-ever I want and tells me stories about everything from mixed martial arts to music videos. Kim bakes cakes and ties banners around the kitchen and sprinkles glittery stars on the worktops to cheer me up. This has a two-fold positive effect. First, it lifts my heart because I love glitter and stars. But second, it makes Cian twitchy to the point of insanity as he can't abide the 'mess'. So even when I'm feeling hideously ill this is stupidly amusing. Yes, we're all very mean to Cian. But he needs to let go and embrace his inner sparkle. Some day ...

I'm acutely aware that my teenagers have had to witness me being horribly sick and unable to get out of bed. It's something that I wish I could shield them from. But that's where the true horror of cancer sticks the knife in and twists it around. I cannot put into words how proud I am of Sacha and Kim. They are kind, considerate and so incredibly caring. I know they worry and I know it's awful for them to see their mother crawling around like a leper, but they have never been anything but supportive. They've had to grow up quickly in many ways. I know my cancer has shattered a certain innocence in them and that makes me sick to my very core. But I have to remind myself, when guilt threatens to choke me, that it's not my fault. I don't want to have cancer and I would do anything in my power to stop it coming back. Instead I have to focus on the fact that I am so lucky to have such amazing young people in my world. I know they will make incredible parents some day – unless their kids dislike glitter and mixed martial arts: then there could be arguments …

The following week I managed to get the second-last chemotherapy session. By now my body was grinding to a halt. My magnesium levels were bottoming out once more so I was prescribed special powders that needed to be taken three times a day. To say that magnesium tastes revolting doesn't begin to describe it. It's like a mixture of metal and petrol with a sweet, sickly aftertaste. I tried mixing it with lots of stuff and settled on cranberry juice as the best thing to mask the flavour. Even still, I had to drink the sachets over the sink because I was retching so violently. I couldn't muster the strength to go for a walk, I could barely eat and I felt disgustingly nauseous all the time. But I was holding on to the thrilling deliciousness that I was nearly there. I was almost across the finishing line.

All the tumours bar one stubborn little bugger on the right-hand side of my neck were gone. So I channelled my energy into the one remaining git. I'd talk to it under my breath (when nobody was listening) and ask it to kindly feck off. I'd bargain with it, letting it know that I'd do something nice for someone less fortunate if it would just leave.

Finally, two weeks later, I pitched up at the hospital, hoping against hope that I would be well enough to endure the last bag of chemotherapy.

The news wasn't great. My bloods were in rag order yet again and the general consensus was that the treatment would need to be held off.

I waited anxiously for David Fennelly to come around. He must've realised I was holding my breath, as he made a deal with me. He'd give me the final treatment on the condition that I returned the following day for a sleepover. I'd need two units of blood and a large bag of magnesium. I would've agreed to anything at that point so I could get it over and done with. It was the weirdest feeling. I was completely and utterly exhausted and knew the final bags of chemotherapy would make me even more nauseous and tired, yet I longed for it to be over. So I sat for the day, falling awkwardly asleep in the chair, with my head-shunting forward and thus waking myself up, as the last dose dripped in. I sincerely hoped it would kill the final tumour without killing me! That evening I drove home and spent the night sweating, tossing and turning as the steroids and other drugs wrangled with my system.

Cian and I were supposed to go to a wedding the following day and my parents were away, so I decided to drive myself to the hospital. That way I could escape as soon as possible when the team allowed me to leave. I had so many kind offers of lifts and I know my friends would've been more than happy to bring me in and collect me again, but I hate having to rely on anyone. I pulled on my pyjamas and got into bed, ready for whatever was thrown at me.

This time the nurses were ready to tackle the magnesium headache. So they gave me Solpadol – the older, tougher cousin of Solapdeine, who takes no prisoners and smashes all pain to pieces. It made things a lot less fractious and the pain in my head was totally manageable.

The blood transfusions began and once more I took a moment to close my eyes and thank the fabulous person who had made the kind donation.

Perhaps it was because my body was totally wrecked or maybe it was due to the fact I'd had so many transfusions, but I felt quite ill during that one. My face, neck and décolletage were flushed and I looked a little like I was sunburnt. I felt woozy and a bit pukey. I think my body was telling me to stay in bed and take it easy.

Cian went to the wedding on his own and I stayed in hospital until early evening. As soon as I was released I did my usual snail-style driving home. Sacha and Kim had lit the fire and were waiting to order takeaway. We watched trash TV and curled up together with Herbie and Tom. There's nothing quite like pets to make you feel relaxed.

The following morning Sacha had a belt test for his kickboxing. Knowing Cian would be out for the count after the wedding, I hauled my ass out of bed. We drove for an hour to the north side of Dublin, where I perched on a high stool, wrapped in a blanket with a headscarf over my balding head, and watched in awe as people kicked and punched one another. It was far more violent than I'd anticipated. But I found it oddly therapeutic. Perhaps the crazy amount of energy being spent was so satisfying to watch because I felt as motivated as a sofa. Afterwards I told Sacha how surprised I was by the level of violence.

'What did you think it would be, Mum?' Sacha asked with a wry smile. 'The clue is in the title: kick – boxing …'

I grinned, knowing I was being utterly stupid. I think I'd convinced myself that there was no contact, just swiping and a bit of jumping around with the odd *urgh* sound effect.

Sacha got his belt and we drove home. I spent the next four days in bed, totally unable to move.

That seemed to be the pattern. If I did anything that required any sort of exertion I was gonzoed and paid the price by having to stay in bed for a few days.

Summer was behind us and Sacha and Kim went back to school. I honestly figured I'd be back swimming in the local pool, going to my office and living life as I had before. But my progress was painfully slow.

I persevered with daily walks, knowing that it was either that or I'd turn into a pumpkin. By that I don't mean to reference Cinderella at midnight: I mean that I'd end up like a round beach ball with a head and limbs.

My weight was at an all-time high. I won't write down what it had risen to because I find it far too depressing. Suffice it to say I wasn't fitting into my clothes and I was tending towards things that were stretchy. Having been a size eight my entire life (bar during my two pregnancies when I was a pie with eyes), it was disconcerting to find myself getting fat. I was barely eating and still putting on weight. In fact, I ate the least amount of food that I can recall. I have a massive appetite and love food but nothing tasted good. Even water had a horrible aftertaste and I found myself not bothering. Chocolate was greasy and tasteless and I couldn't bear coffee. I drank no alcohol and was more able to stomach fruit than sweets. So by rights, I should've been Twiggy's twin. But instead I was more like Benny Hill. Not fair.

A month after the chemotherapy finished, I realised my hearing was going downhill. I was constantly asking people to speak up or repeat what they'd said. It sounded as if I had a bucket over my head and I was getting headaches and finding the constant need to strain a burden. I was watching TV at a sound level that frightened the dog so I figured I'd better go back to Aoife and have another audio test.

This time as I sat in the *Mr & Mrs* soundproof booth in the big red chair things weren't quite so fabulous. The computer read-out confirmed what I already knew – my hearing was badly affected. I went to see Mr Glynn the ENT specialist to see what he thought of the situation.

My only hope of reversal was to try steroids. First I had to take a decreasing oral dose – starting with twelve steroids the first day, ten the second and so on. Meanwhile I was fitted with hearing aids. Unlike the large lump of custard-coloured plastic with a huge contraption inside the ear I'd seen years ago, my little ones were practically invisible and, marvellously, I was able to hear. It's not the same as having the hearing restored, but it's a damn sight better than nothing.

For the first week I could hear the toilet flushing from a mile away and it sounded like Niagara Falls. Putting plates in the dishwasher was ear shattering and sounded as if there was a large lump hammer in the equation. Scrunching up a piece of paper was like metal being crushed by a large machine.

But Aoife assured me that my brain would adjust and learn to block out background noise while focusing on voices and the things I needed to hear.

The actual devices took a little bit of getting used to. I wasn't great, I realised, at shoving small objects all the way inside my ear. We're conditioned into being careful while using a cotton bud to clean and never to push it in too far. So this went against the grain for me at the start. But a whole new world had opened up to me. I hadn't realised how badly my hearing had been affected until it had improved again. I'd stopped talking to people while out and about – the person at the cash desk in the supermarket or other dog walkers. It was too embarrassing to have to say, 'Sorry? Pardon? Apologies – can you repeat that?' So I'd slightly retreated without knowing.

I now have a whole new empathy for the hard of hearing. I never imagined it was an easy obstacle to overcome but now I know for sure that it's really difficult.

After two weeks I returned to the audio suite to see if there was any improvement. Sadly, there wasn't. I saw Fergal Glynn again and he explained that the only possible option open to me was steroid injections into the inner ear.

'How is that done?' I asked, wincing at the very thought of it. Fergal explained that he'd put in some local anaesthetic and then he'd burst the ear drum with a needle and inject steroid solution inside.

'So I'd be awake?' I said. He nodded.

Mr Glynn said it might be a little uncomfortable. I did point out that many moons ago my gynaecologist had told me that having a baby without an epidural might be uncomfortable too … He laughed.

There was a downside – apart from the obviously awful procedure: there was less than a ten per cent chance of it working.

What had happened was that those tiny hairs inside the ear that are responsible for making us hear had, in the end, been obliterated by the chemotherapy. Fergal explained that there are two main ways these tiny hairs can be damaged. Either by a viral infection, such as measles, or by chemicals. I fell into the chemical bracket and the results after chemical damage weren't positive. So I could end up with a hole in each eardrum (that mightn't heal) and copious amounts of ear infections going forward.

'If it was you, and your ears were in the same shape as mine, would you do it?' I asked.

'No,' he said honestly. 'I wouldn't. I don't think it's worth the risk. I don't think it'll work. But it's up to you.'

I sat and pondered for a while and made the decision to quit while I was ahead. The hearing aids were helping massively and I was managing. I didn't need to end up in a situation where I had ongoing ear infections. I had enough crap on my plate, thank you very much.

So I walked out of Fergal's office that day satisfied I'd made the right decision for me.

Another lump had appeared on the left side of my neck. So I had two that needed to be obliterated. It would've been lovely to know I was cancer free after all I'd been through. But I had to accept that most of the tumours had been tackled. I'd partially lost my hearing along the way, but even if I'd known it was going to happen, I would have gone ahead with the treatment. Most of the cancer was gone and that was good enough for me.

Knowing that there were a few nodes still hanging around, Dr Fennelly needed for me to have a PET scan. Sadly, and this can happen a lot, the insurance company refused to fund it.

But St David had another thing up his sleeve. A brand new test that uses a tiny biopsy from the patient to precisely match the right targeted therapy for that person. The advantages of this test are mind blowing. Because treatments are targeted for each patient the outcomes will be improved. For cases like mine where I've used up a lot of options, this test will find the drugs best suited to me. For patients who are newly diagnosed, it will give your oncologist a clear picture of what you should be using, removing any uncertainty.

I had my test carried out in the UK with a company called Oncologica and their test is called Oncofocus. I think it's one of the best advances I've seen in oncology. This cuts out the awful disappointment of being put on chemotherapy and finding it doesn't work. It's also scientific, which always gives me great comfort.

So my sample was sent away and they promised to have results in ten days. Dr Fennelly mentioned PARP inhibitors as his guess for me.

Apparently there are two new PARP inhibitors coming through the pipelines. So perhaps one of them will suit me. If one works for me, it could mean that this will be the last time I have to deal with cancer. It could mean that there is something that I can take orally that will give me my life back – back to the way it was before 2005 when the BRCA1 gene came crashing into my life, bringing cancer with it.

My results were in from the Oncofocus test. They had kindly offered to send them to me by email at the same time as Dr Fennelly. I eagerly used the special password they'd given to open the document.

Cian and I sat like two little bunnies waiting to read it through. It was very colourful and there were several pages, but none of it was remotely intelligible to us, the non-oncologists. After a few minutes I asked Cian gingerly, 'So do you get what they're saying?'

'Not a word,' he said as we fell around laughing. Luckily Dr Fennelly was able to read all of it and even commented on how precise and interesting it was. We nodded.

'We haven't a clue what any of it says,' I said, letting him know we weren't even going to pretend.

So he explained that it had told us all the things we'd found out along the way over the ten years. It detected that I'm a positive carrier of the BRCA 1 gene. It knew I have breast cancer and that it's triple negative. But most importantly it threw out a few treatments that would work for me. It was Christmas so I went home to my six Christmas trees and a house covered in glitter and tinsel.

Christmas was a washout as I had to troop in and out of hospital due to an infection and for pain management. The two remaining tumours had been joined by a third and they were sitting on the nerves leading into my shoulder, neck and right arm. I spent ten days in hospital in late January of 2017 while the wonderful nurses tried to help with the pain. Missy, the pain specialist, was fantastic and reassured me that this would be transient. I had everything from electric shock treatment (yes that still happens in 2017!) to steroid injections to my shoulder to try and kill the pain. But it became clear nothing was going to work fully.

You see, we were waiting to hear if I would be given a drug that was still on trial. It was the golden egg that my oncofocus test had suggested. There was a lot of paperwork and phone calls and I knew it wasn't going to be a speedy process.

The next couple of months threw a lot in my direction. I tried another type of tablet that didn't work either. I ended up in hospital for ten days as the pain team tried to curb my nerve pain. All the while, the cancer continued to grow. I was at a very low ebb when I met with a genetic oncology specialist called Professor David Gallagher. Along with David (yes I know there are many Davids, my apologies) Fennelly, they came up with another chemotherapy to try. I now have a few treatments under my belt. The pain is ebbing away and so too are the nasty tumours.

I'm slowly crawling out of the dark hole of sickness and pain. I'm out walking as often as I can; Herbie is always up for a walk and he lifts my spirits sky high when I see his happy face.

I'm back doing smoothies. This time with the NutriBullet. Why did nobody tell me about this gadget? I know there are a million adverts on TV for it all the time, but someone should've stopped me in the street and asked 'have you got a NutriBullet yet? Why not? You need one.'

I started with a masticator and moved on to the super-di-dooper juicer, and even faster again is this fella. Peel the fruit, bung it in, add some rice, milk or juice, it makes a loud grinding noise and, hey presto, the whole family has a smoothie.

Cian and I are *very* enthusiastic about it. Sacha is good at taking his, seeing as he won't eat breakfast. Kim is the most resistant. But I'll break her down, don't you worry.

I'm hoping this new chemotherapy will kill the cancer I've got now. Science says it will. So that gives me massive hope. Dr Fennelly and his team are continuing their quest to find me a PARP inhibitor that doesn't make me vomit repeatedly. He believes they are the way to go. If there's one out there that will help, I know St David will find it.

I intend getting back into all my clothes again someday too. I can see the real me in the distance. I'm waving to her and I'm beckoning her to come forth. I know that better times are ahead. I have so much fluffy hair that I have an appointment with the hairdresser's tomorrow!

Work is great. I have a clatter of loyal readers who jolly me along on Twitter (@MsEmmaHannigan) and Facebook (Author Emma Hannigan) and via my website (www.emmahannigan.com). I know I have many, many people rooting for me and that's a wonderful feeling.

My next novel is finished. I'm moving my mind onto what I'll write next. I adore the deliciousness of exploring what the new characters will be like and who they'll love or loathe.

My husband and children are healthy. My parents are travelling the world and refusing to retire from either work or life. They're dead right.

I hope that medicine continues to make huge leaps forward and that the research that has begun will produce new and better cancer treatments. I hope that more patients survive and that fewer families have to bear the sadness of loss.

If I had one wish, it would be that cancer no longer existed. It's the most cruel and hideous disease. I despise it. But for as long as I have breath in my body I will continue to fight back. I will continue to write and talk about it just in case my story happens to help someone else.

At the beginning of this book I said that when I was first diagnosed I looked for a book written in plain English that would give me hope. If I've done that for anybody reading this, then my job is done.

I don't know what the future holds for me. But then again, neither does anyone else! Until I'm told not to, I'll keep on going. Of course, I secretly hope that there's a PARP inhibitor waiting in the wings to change my health and perhaps give me some more time. After all, if I don't dream, I've no chance of those dreams coming true.

Never in a million years had I imagined way back in 2005, when my cancer journey began, that I would wind up being an author, keynote speaker, or ambassador or on TV and radio. It's all totally bananas.

Of course I'm not glad I got cancer. But I appreciate the life I've carved for myself since being diagnosed. There is more hope than ever that cancer will change from being a potentially deadly illness to a chronic condition that can be managed over long periods of time.

I cannot even begin to guess how long I have left to live. I don't really go there in my head. But, hey, we're all terminal – right? What I can tell you, with full confidence, is that I am grateful for the years my treatment has bought me. I am grateful that the type of cancer I get is sensitive to treatments and that it has gone away each time thus far.

I have come around to accepting that cancer will always be a part of my life. It is what it is. As long as medicine can keep up with my diagnoses, I'm safe. I am crossing my fingers and toes it does.

Many years ago Dr David Fennelly told me to let him worry about the medical part while I got on with my life. I took his word as gospel and I try to do just as he suggested.

I'm grateful for so much, but most of all I'm grateful for the fact I'm still here and in a position to enjoy my life. I'd forgive you for believing my life revolves solely around cancer, considering that's what I've focused on in this book. But there are many lovely things that invade my thoughts. Things that are nothing to do with hospitals, things that give me joy. I'm a very happy person and I honestly feel I have a great life.

I'm not bitter or angry. I don't feel I have anything to be angry about.

All I can do is take each day as it comes and do my best to roll with the punches when they hurtle towards me. I do see myself being on this earth long enough to grow old. I want to be that lady in Jenny Joseph's poem 'Warning' who wears purple. I love this poem and it makes me smile every time I read it. I have already embraced the 'purple' inside me. No matter what life throws at me from here on in, I'll try my very best to meet it head on.

If you've just been diagnosed with cancer, or if you know someone who has, I'd like you to take hope and positivity from my story. Survival rates are climbing all the time. Fight the good fight and, who knows, maybe you'll find yourself winning like I am.

Onwards and upwards, folks!

Love and light,

Emma x

Some Extra Information

As I mentioned before there are various stages of cancer – here's a quick rundown which might be useful.

Many of us will have heard of the 'stages' of cancer. The stage of cancer is based on the size of the tumour. The purpose of the staging system is to help the doctors to sort the different factors and some of the 'personality' features of the cancer into categories. There a number of reasons for this:

1. So the doctor and patient can best understand the prognosis (the most likely outcome of the disease).

2. So the medical team have a guide for treatment decisions (together with other parts of your pathology/lab reports). Many clinical studies of breast cancer treatments that you and your doctor will consider are partly organised by the staging system.

3. To help provide a common way to describe the extent of cancer present. All doctors and nurses the world over use 'staging' as a universal system and language when discussing cancer. This means that oncologists, doctors and nurses can use the results of their patients' treatments for comparison purposes. All the while, this can aid the ongoing development of treatments and successful outcomes with patients.

Here are the main stages of cancer and what each one usually indicates. It is important to note that I am referring to breast cancer, as that is what I've experienced. This is also a guide in my own words. I am obviously not an oncologist and I'm also blonde, so this is simply a 'plain English' guide!

Stage 0

Stage 0 is used to describe non-invasive breast cancers, such as DCIS and LCIS. In stage 0, there is no evidence of cancer cells or non-cancerous abnormal cells breaking out of the part of the breast in which they started, or of getting through to or invading neighbouring normal tissue. This is what I would have had at the time of my mastectomy. In a nutshell, the pre-cancer cells appeared to have remained intact in the area of tissue that I had removed.

Stage I

Stage I describes invasive breast cancer (cancer cells are breaking through to or invading neighbouring normal tissue). Two points are vital with Stage I:

1. The tumour measures up to 2 centimetres, and

2. No surrounding lymph nodes are involved.

Stage II

Stage II is divided into two subcategories, called IIA and IIB.
    Stage IIA describes invasive breast cancer with these characteristics:

1. No tumour or lump can be found in the breast, but cancer cells are found in the axillary lymph nodes (the lymph nodes under the arm – essentially, the area where we all put deodorant), or

2. The tumour measures 2 centimetres or less and has spread to the axillary lymph nodes, or

3. The tumour is larger than 2 centimetres but not larger than 5 centimetres and has not spread to the axillary lymph nodes.

Stage IIB describes invasive breast cancer in which:

1. The tumour is larger than 2 but no larger than 5 centimetres and has spread to the axillary lymph nodes, or

2. The tumour is larger than 5 centimetres but has not spread to the axillary lymph nodes.

Stage III

Stage III is divided into three subcategories: IIIA, IIIB and IIIC.

Stage IIIA describes invasive breast cancer in which one of the following has happened:

1. No tumour is found in the breast. But cancer is found in axillary lymph nodes that are clumped together or sticking to other structures. The cancer may have spread to lymph nodes near the breastbone, or

2. The tumour is 5 centimetres or smaller and has spread to axillary lymph nodes that are clumped together or sticking to other structures, or

3. The tumour is larger than 5 centimetres and has spread to axillary lymph nodes that are clumped together or sticking to other structures.

Stage IIIB describes invasive breast cancer in which one of the following has happened:

1. The tumour may be any size and has spread to the chest wall and/or skin of the breast, and

2. The cancer may also have spread to axillary lymph nodes that are clumped together or sticking to other structures. Or the cancer may have spread to lymph nodes near the breastbone.

Stage IIIC describes invasive breast cancer in which one or all of the following scenarios may occur:

1. There may be no sign of cancer, in the actual breast. Or, if there is a tumour, it may be any size and may have spread to the chest wall and/or the skin of the breast, and

2. The cancer has spread to lymph nodes above or below the collarbone, and

3. The cancer may have spread to axillary lymph nodes or to lymph nodes near the breastbone.

Stage IV

Stage IV describes invasive breast cancer where:

1. The cancer has spread to other organs of the body. Often the lungs, liver, bones or brain.

'Metastatic at presentation' means that the breast cancer has spread beyond the breast and nearby lymph nodes, even though this is the first diagnosis of breast cancer. The reason for this is that the 'primary' or first part of the breast cancer was not found when it was only inside the breast. Metastatic cancer is considered Stage IV.

Additional staging information

You may also hear terms such as 'early' or 'earlier' stage, 'later' or 'advanced' stage breast cancer. Unlike the 'staging' system, these terms are not medically precise.

Some doctors may use these words differently. As I mentioned at the beginning of this chapter, I am obviously not an oncologist, so don't quote me on this, but I hope that this might shed a little light on the general idea of how those words can apply to the official staging system.

Early stage
Stage 0
Stage I
Stage II
Some stage III

Later or advanced stage
Other stage III
Stage IV

It's important to keep in mind that just because you are told you have Stage 0 or even Stage IV you still don't have my permission to go and buy that shovel! No digging your own grave. No giving in or giving up is allowed. There is always hope. There is never time to give up fighting the good fight.

Here are some websites you might find useful:

www.cancer.ie
www.cancerbuddiesnetwork.org
www.arcccancersupport.ie
www.cancerresearchuk.org
www.macmillan.org.uk
www.cancerscreening.nhs.uk

Top Tips for Getting Through Treatment!

Beauty is only skin deep ...

It has never mattered to me how attractive or classically good-looking a person may be deemed: it's what's inside that really matters. I know plenty of strikingly beautiful people who don't float my boat because they aren't particularly pleasant. As a matter of fact, once I get to know a person, it makes no odds to me what they look like either way. But I would be lying if I said my own appearance doesn't concern or interest me. I've pondered this and I've come to the conclusion that it's not entirely a vanity thing either. I'm covered in scars, I have a broken nose, false boobs and I detest my thighs, so I'm hardly a perfect specimen. But for me, there is a direct correlation between looking good and feeling better.

I trained as a beauty therapist because I loved the idea of working with people to make them feel good about themselves too. I love connecting with others and if I wasn't such a wuss I might have opted for nursing. But, hand on heart, I couldn't do that job. I'd be useless. So I went for the more pampering part of caring.

My training has saved me a fortune in waxing, manicures and facials, but after the initial few years, I haven't used my training commercially. I often thought of the money I'd spent on my course, and indeed the hours of study to get my grades, and felt it was a pity I hadn't utilised it better.

When cancer came crashing into my life and my outward image changed radically and I was left looking like a different person, I channelled my training. All of a sudden the time and energy didn't seem wasted.

On the days when I was bald and had that hideous chemotherapy pallor, my knowledge of skin care, make-up and general grooming helped me to look and feel more 'normal'.

Listed below are the things that I've found invaluable over the years. I'm hoping that one or two might resonate with you and make you feel better too!

Eyebrow tattooing

This might sound like a drastic move, but once you find a reputable tattoo artist it'll change your opinion! There's no rule that you need to be a cancer patient to get this done either. I would recommend this to everyone. It's a fantastic cheat for framing the face.

My eyebrows grew back as best they could after my multiple treatments but, despite their earnest efforts, they were a bit sad looking. They were spiky and patchy and a bit like two malnourished and pecked-at caterpillars. I always needed to add to them with an eyebrow pencil. I don't know how deft you are with one of those, but depending on how rushed I was in the mornings, the results varied. Some days they looked great, others they were either on the skinny side – or indeed the poor caterpillars transformed into two fat slugs.

I've seen some dreadful eyebrow tattooing that made the victim look as if a toddler had been at their face with an indelible marker. So make sure you ask the tattoo artist for some before and after photos of their work.

I was fortunate to meet Elizabeth Oakes (www.elizabethoakes.ie). She works in Ireland, the UK, the US and the Middle East. In short, she is the *grand dame* of permanent make-up. She has even designed her own hand tool for grafting tattooed eyebrows onto grateful ladies' faces.

She recommends two sessions to achieve the perfect arch. I cannot believe the difference my new eyebrows have made. They really do frame my face shape and I'm amazed by how much better that makes me feel. Instead of feeling like I've been left with dodgy tufts, I am now the envy of my friends! This treatment lasts for years too, so even though it may seem like a big outlay at first, it's a sound investment. Who doesn't want to wake up looking ready to go? Elizabeth also trains people to become permanent-make-up artists, so if you're looking for a new venture you could go along to one of her workshops. Believe me, I'm very tempted! I know I'd have a line of friends looking for new brows. Having said that, I'm struggling to find enough hours in the day as it is … Maybe I'll leave it to the expert after all!

Incidentally, Elizabeth also does areola tattooing for women who've had a mastectomy. I've seen the results first hand and they are astonishing.

Wigs and hairpieces

Many women going through chemotherapy and radiation lose their hair. This is usually a temporary side effect and in most cases the hair will grow back with a vengeance – literally as soon as the treatment finishes. I know only too well how it feels when your hair starts to thin. Everything gets covered in shedding hair and, before long, patches of scalp begin to shine through like pale, mocking beacons of unwanted light. This can be a heartbreaking time for anybody, male or female. But all I can say is that you need to try to keep in mind that this is transient and you will be back to your old self before long.

Hair loss is a weird thing. Let's face it, women never think it'll happen to them. It's hardly something we plan or wish for. But it's more common than we realise. Many people suffer with alopecia, which is often a permanent problem requiring a more permanent solution.

Some choose to rock the bald look. A great tip I've heard of for those women is to use a blusher brush and some dark-brown eye shadow to dust the head, creating a false hairline to give the illusion of hair and also define the head and forehead.

But in my own experience, I wanted to avoid looking bald. I felt it was too much of a neon sign to strangers that I was having cancer treatment. (Obviously I don't actually see myself as being sick at all, so therefore I don't want to look it either!)

As I outlined earlier, back in 2007 the yokes on offer were enough to make me depressed. Happily things have moved forward and changed for the better. My favourite place for either wigs or hairpieces is called the Hair Club (www.hairclub.ie) in Ireland or Hot Hair (www.hothair.co.uk) in England. If you look online there are a whole host of trendy looks on offer.

During my last course of radiation treatment I lost all the hair from the back of my head only. I found a brilliantly clever strip of hair that clipped in easily, and in a matter of seconds I was back to normal. By the way, if you need a wonderful ponytail or some extensions to bulk up your natural hair these places are wonderful for that too. Not a deceased animal in sight – I promise!

If wigs are not for you, there are many places offering specifically designed hats for people with hair loss. Unlike normal hats, these come down lower at the back and cover all the areas where hair would normally be.

You're never fully dressed without a smile ...

Smiling is a marvellous thing. After all, a smile is the prettiest thing a girl can wear! On days when I felt low and under the weather I used to practise smiling in the mirror. Try it – just don't get caught or you could be arrested!

Lipstick is fantastic for lifting the complexion. During treatment we all need any help we can get. I opt for a strong rather than pale colour. I adore deep reds or magenta pinks and they always make me feel happier. If you're not a lipstick queen, wean yourself onto them by choosing a moisturising gloss.

Post-mastectomy lingerie – no booby prizes here!

One of the most depressing moments I ever had involved a hideous bra.

If you're around my age (early forties) or older, you will remember the unattractive and dreadfully uncomfortable bras that were on offer in the eighties. This was well before Eva Herzigova made us all pea-green with envy in her 'Hello Boys' billboard commercial campaign for the relaunch of the Wonderbra. And unless you were in a position to afford La Perla, the general Josephine Soaps among us were wearing heavily constructed contraptions – over-the-shoulder-boulder-holders that were, in a word, awful.

Times have moved on and, thankfully, most large chain stores and fashion outlets stock pretty and appealing bras that women of all ages, shapes and sizes can enjoy feeling pretty in.

When I chose to have a bilateral mastectomy in 2006 I had no qualms about the surgery and was truly relieved once it was over.

But the post-mastectomy underwear that I encountered just after that surgery was a blow I wasn't expecting. Like the eighties monstrosities, they had hard, scratchy half-lace half-slippy nylon cups and straps so thick they looked as if they could be used for towing large vehicles. It baffled and upset me that anyone felt the need to make them look so bloody ugly. The icing on the cake – or, in this instance, the poo on the shoe – was that they were eye-wateringly expensive. They were, excuse the pun, the booby prize of lingerie.

I actually dreaded putting these bras on. In my own head I felt like some sort of fashion outcast. I know you could argue that nobody could see these things – and believe me nobody saw them! But knowing they were there, lurking like monsters beneath my clothes, was enough to make me frown.

I missed going to the lingerie sections of high-street stores and picking up the odd bra-and-pants set. I felt I'd been banished to the nasty bra club forever.

I still remember the day I found an entire nest of post-surgery bras in my local M&S! At that moment, all that was missing was a beacon of shining light from above and dramatic drum-rolling music. For the first time in years I wasn't an outsider. And the prices! I'd forgotten how fabulous it was to be in a position to pay high-street prices. Since that day I have been an avid M&S-underwear wearer. Their range can be bought online too (in Ireland at www.marksandspencer.ie or in the UK at www.marksandspencer.com).

Debenhams (www.debenhams.ie in Ireland or www.debenhams.com in the UK) are also fantastic and they offer a really good fitting service as well.

I'm sure, just like the improvements in wigs, there are many amazing new websites selling non-offensive post-surgery underwear nowadays, but I adore the notion that I too can shop in 'normal' stores again!

Incidentally, there is a superb range of post-surgery bras for women recovering from mastectomy by a company called Theya Lingerie (www.theyalingerie.com). These products are made from bamboo, which is ultra soft and far more absorbent than cotton – fantastic for menopausal women. In addition, bamboo has antiseptic properties which makes it perfect for healing skin. The designers have gone to great lengths to ensure these bras are user friendly for post-op ladies. Some fasten to the front to avoid twisting and uncomfortable wriggling, and the labels are all printed onto the fabric so there's no worry of anything digging into sensitive skin. They are quite functional-looking at first glance, but the comfort level overrides the initial impression. Also, I was incredibly surprised by how neat and invisible they are under clothing, even tight vest tops. They have removable padding so they work brilliantly if you are waiting for reconstruction.

Theya Lingerie also do a line of pants that come up higher than usual, which would be a welcome blessing for women who've had reconstruction using fat from the abdominal area. In this instance, the healing properties of the bamboo material is a stroke of genius. These pants are streamlined too, so there's very little VPL involved.

MLD

I mentioned MLD, or manual lymphatic drainage, in a previous chapter and it was the answer to my prayers. Be certain that the practitioner you choose is properly qualified. If possible he or she should be a chartered physiotherapist with lots of oncology experience. Don't go for someone who did a weekend course and thinks they know it all. They could injure you further.

I believe I found the jewel in the crown when it comes to MLD. Deborah Fernandes is clinical director of Physiofit Woman in Sandyford, Dublin (www.physiofitwoman.ie). She is a chartered physiotherapist as well as being trained in the Leduc method of MLD.

When done properly, I cannot recommend this treatment highly enough. Always check with your doctor that it is safe for you to have this before you begin.

This treatment is generally suitable for anyone who has had surgery. I had a mole removed from my foot and ended up with an elephantised ankle – I had MLD and it was sorted.

Reflexology

I swear by reflexology. Again there are many therapists out there and I urge you to research and ensure the one you choose is actually qualified to treat oncology patients. I went to several who were perfectly lovely human beings but not great therapists. My reflex-ologist, Michelle, is a registered nurse and knows her stuff. She studied specific oncology reflexology modules and is one of those women I instantly put my trust in.

Reflexology helps to flush toxins from the body while promoting natural healing. It's also incredibly relaxing and aids sleep and relieves stress. Who doesn't need that? If you're suffering from bowel issues as a result of treatment, this is wonderful for relieving the symptoms. I don't do many alternative treatments, and I'm very wary of ingesting anything that isn't medically approved, but reflexology is totally safe and after four years of regular treatments I know it helps me. By the way, it's not obligatory to have cancer. Reflexology is wonderful for anybody and is especially brilliant for pregnant ladies or people with fertility problems.

This is also a lovely treatment for partners or family members of a person going through cancer. I cannot imagine how difficult it must be to sit by and watch someone you love struggling with illness. This is a stress-busting treat that can only benefit the client.

Tanning – the only safe way is to fake it

Skin is ultra-sensitive to sunlight during cancer treatment. Sunburn is not something you want to add to your troubles. I don't sit in the sun ever, but I am descended from the Smurfs and am almost blue in colour, so the sun and I were never going to be friends. If you're in the throes of treatment or you naturally sport a very pale complexion, you are probably a bit of a fake-tan fan.

I am a master when it comes to fake tan – even if I say so myself. I stumbled upon Tan Organic and they offer a range of products that are free from chemicals and parabens. That's obviously great news for all of us. But of their entire range, the one thing that really floats my boat is the self-tanning oil. It has got to be one of the most amazing inventions, especially for dry or sensitive skin types. This is so easy to use I figured there must be a catch – but there isn't! It comes in a lovely glass bottle and all you have to do is apply it to your skin after a shower. It doubles up as a moisturiser, so instead of having that slightly scaly look some fake-tan products can cause, this leaves a lovely dewy glow. It's applied with your bare hands so no mitts or gloves are required. I use it after my swim and simply clean my hands with a baby wipe to remove any residue from my palms.

During chemotherapy and radiation most of us suffer with uber-dry skin. This isn't normal dryness: this is a chemical dehydration that can leave skin feeling tight, itchy and, from personal experience, a bit reptile-like. Tan Organic self-tanning oil has literally been my skin saviour. The best part is that it actually smells pleasant too. What's not to love? It's widely stocked or you can buy it at www.tanorganic. com.

Another go-to tanning product is Cocoa Brown by Marissa Carter. This one is also paraben free and has the incredible plus of coming in a one-hour version. This mousse (which comes in normal or darker shades) is also very easy to apply using a mitt and gives a long-lasting effect that fades really well. It's available from Primark and is certainly not a bank buster.

If you're looking for a luxury brand, my favourite is Fake Bake. Yet again this one is free from parabens. Ask for it at your local salon too. In my opinion it's the best spray tan I've ever had. If I'm going to something special I always opt for Fake Bake at my local salon. It's a good one for going on holiday too, as it fades well. No scaly patches or dark-orange tide marks.

My original favourite, and I still buy it the odd time, is St. Tropez. They have a new product called St. Tropez Gradual Tan in Shower Golden Glow. It does as the name suggests – you simply rub it on in the shower, wait three minutes and wash it off. I find this product good, but I know when I was feeling dreadful there was no way I could've stood wet and cold in the shower for three minutes. So maybe this is one for the days when you're feeling a bit better.

No matter which product you decide on, and it's best to try a few to see which one best suits your own complexion, it's worth avoiding ones with harsh chemicals and parabens. After all, our skin is our largest organ and we shouldn't lather it in nasties.

Nail it!
During chemotherapy my previously strong and long nails became brittle and weak. They began to peel off in scales. Wow, this cancer

thing isn't attractive, is it? If this is happening to you, don't panic! Sally Hansen is here to rescue us like a knight with a shining bottle. Out of the hundreds of nail-conditioning and strengthening products on the market, ranging in price from cheap as chips to bank-bustingly dear, my favourite and the one I found most effective is called Miracle Nail Thickener – it comes in a purple bottle with a gold lid. I was quite diligent and applied it twice daily for a week. It worked wonders for my flaky nails and I always make sure I use it in between manicures to keep my nails healthy.

The other failsafe option is to use a cuticle oil. These are available in all pharmacies and supermarkets. Almond oil and olive oil are both highly effective too. Soak a cotton-wool pad with either, dab it generously onto the nails and cuticles and leave to soak in. Incidentally, olive oil works wonders on the skin too. My only reservation with that one is that I feel a little bit like I've been working over a deep-fat fryer!

If you've ended up with unsightly white ridges on your nails you might feel happier with a two-week manicure. Check it out with your own oncologist, but my team have no issue with me having Shellac or a similar manicure done. It can be a lovely way to add a splash of colour to your hands and give you a pretty boost. To avoid dried-out cuticles or nails apply a generous slick of cuticle oil each night before you go to bed. It really helps to save your nails and stop them from being like dried-out paper when the Shellac comes off.

Mouth ulcers – what a pain!

If you're in the midst of radiation or chemotherapy and you're getting mouth ulcers or radiation burns inside your mouth, I feel your pain. When you're already feeling lousy from the treatment, it can feel like the final straw when a throbbing, eye-wateringly painful mouth ulcer joins in and adds to the misery.

Many treatments are available either over the counter (Kin is my favourite mouthwash) or on prescription, but the absolute star of the show for me is a little home remedy. All you need is a glass of tepid water (cold water is too shocking to the delicate surface in your mouth) and a tablespoon of old-fashioned bread soda.

Mix the two together, stand over the sink, gargle and swirl the mixture around in your mouth and then spit it out. Repeat until the glass is empty. You want to feel a slight sandy or gritty texture coating the inside of your mouth. This is not the most attractive thing to do and shouldn't be done in front of anyone you're trying to impress, but believe me, it works. It is brilliant for radiation burns on the hard palate or any kind of nasty ulcers. Do it three or even four times a day until the symptoms are relieved. It's magical and, hey, if you get really good at aiming there are lots of competitions in parts of the US where you can win good money for spitting …

If your throat is sore, swallow a tiny amount of the liquid. The gritty mixture will help with healing.

Vaginal dryness

This is an issue that can cause real discomfort for so many women, especially during chemotherapy. It's essential to try and avoid gels or creams that might contain perfume. My go-to product is by a company called Multi-Gyn. Their ActiGel helps treat vaginal dryness and discomfort. It's safe to use every day and can be a godsend if you're feeling itchy and sore.

Nausea

I am a strong believer in asking for anti-sickness medication. The best one I've ever used is a three-day course called Emend. This is taken on the day of chemotherapy and for two days afterwards.

For general sickness I find Motilium fantastic. Stemetil is another good one. When I was really ill my saviour was Valoid.

But once you've been prescribed the right drugs by your medical team, it is possible to help yourself too. Eating is vital. I know it can seem like an impossible task to eat when you know your poor tummy is like a washing machine, but lining the stomach always helps. Dry crackers with a cup of weak Bovril is a good one to start with. I found soup to be a good thing to eat at times too. If you can make your own, all the better.

Sucking on boiled sweets helped me on occasion too. In fact, a wonderfully kind lady by the name of Margaret Divilly sent me a box of special sweets called Queasy Drops. They're boiled sweets in flavours such as sour cherry and were a real help when I was at my worst. These can be bought online and make a lovely gift for someone who is ill.

Ice pops can be easier to take than solid foods and I often freeze fresh juices to make healthier snacks.

But in my experience the key to avoiding really terrible nausea is to eat small amounts more often. So sticking to three square meals a day mightn't work, but try to have something small every couple of hours instead.

If you're feeling really dreadful, try sipping iced water for a few minutes and then try to eat a cream cracker or a rice cake. Once your stomach takes a little food on board it's easier to try something else.

Nutrition
I've done all sorts of diets over the years in the hope that they would stop the cancer from returning. None of them has worked.

I know there are lots of people who swear by certain diets but in my case I am finally resting easily with the notion that eating sensibly and healthily is where it's at. I avoid processed foods and try to keep sugar, dairy and gluten to a minimum.

Cancer treatment can wreak havoc with most patients' diets. Whether it's down to nausea or being neutropenic, many of us have to change some aspects of what we eat during treatment. Similar to during pregnancy, there are some no-nos when it comes to what we eat.

For example, if a patient is neutropenic and therefore in danger of picking up infections easily, it's not advisable to eat too much raw food or unpasteurised cheese or shellfish. It's mostly down to common sense, but always take advice from your caregiver. When prone to infection, it's best to minimise the risk of food poisoning or having an upset stomach.

If you're feeling utterly dreadful and can't stomach eating your usual meals, it can help to change things a little to suit. It'll only be for a while, so don't worry about never being able to eat 'normally' ever again. It will pass and you will be able to get back to eating foie gras and buttered lobster (if that's your preference) once treatment ends.

I tend to struggle the most at breakfast time – with nausea, the thought of my usual porridge doesn't appeal. So on the days when it looks more like a bowl of frog spawn than a nourishing breakfast, I mix up a smoothie. Often liquid is easier on the tummy than solids. There's no right or wrong way to make a smoothie. All you need is a blender and a juicer.

I spent a fortune on a high-grade masticator back in the day. This is a slow juicer that is said to preserve most of the vitamins and nutrients of the fruits and vegetables. I've no doubt that masticators do that indeed. But, dear Lord, they take ages. They are a chore to clean and by the time you have enough juice to work with, you've lost the will to live altogether.

If you don't have an extra hour in the morning, or indeed if you have my low level of patience, I'd recommend the Sage Juicer or a Nutribullet. Far faster, with less fuss, and if one or two vitamins or minerals are lost in the process, I can live with that.

For a nourishing breakfast smoothie I typically use whatever fruit is in season. I'm not a fan of using blueberries in winter, as they taste like battery acid and are wildly expensive. So try to use whatever is on special offer in the local shop. That means it's not breaking the bank and you can be pretty certain it's in season so therefore at its best. Below are a couple of ideas, but if you'd like some further recipes I'd recommend Jason Vale's books. I've not sure if it's partly psychological, but I feel so much better since I've been juicing. I've had very few colds and my general health has improved.

A great juice that's packed with antioxidants and good immune-system-boosting stuff is a mixture of carrot, beetroot and orange. It tastes delicious and is a good one for fussy kids. Another favourite in our house is pineapple, apple, lime, pear and spinach. I know that sounds like it could be vile, but believe me it's not! Drinking juices regularly isn't going to eradicate the world of cancer, but it does promote good general health and I know it certainly doesn't do any harm.

Juice of 1 apple
Juice of 1 orange
Juice of ½ lime

1 handful of spinach leaves
½ banana
½ cup dry porridge oats
2 generous tablespoons of mixed seeds (they can be bought premixed in all supermarkets)
½ cup of yoghurt
Glug of honey or squirt of maple or agave syrup to taste

During summer I would throw in a handful of berries such as raspberries, blueberries, blackberries, strawberries etc. There are no hard and fast rules to this. Pineapple is another lovely fruit to add, but make sure it's nice and ripe.

First use your juicer to extract your juice and then put it in a liquidiser or blender or NutriBullet with all the other ingredients and whizz it up. What comes out is a lovely, thick milk-shake-type consistency. It doesn't need to be downed in one. If you're feeling awful, sip it over the morning. But it will line your stomach and I usually feel a whole lot better once I get some of this into my tummy. If you're feeling really retchy and ill, take an anti-nausea tablet, wait fifteen minutes and then try some.

Don't forget to wash the spinach first. But this is a really good way of getting greens and iron into your ailing body. It won't taste like you're eating a load of grass either, I promise!

I don't eat much dairy, so I tend to use soya yoghurt, but you can choose whatever flavour or type you like.

Soup is another thing that I eat a lot. Homemade soup is incredibly nourishing and easy to digest, so learning to make your own is a skill that will stand to you. It can be a perfectly balanced meal, depending on what you put in. On days when you feel you can't bear to eat a plate of solid food, this can be a godsend.

All soups can be made using this simple base.

1 onion
2 potatoes
3 cups of stock
1 cup of chopped carrot

1 cup of chopped parsnip
1 cup of chopped leeks
1 cooked chicken breast
Salt and pepper to season

Peel and chop the onion and potatoes – make sure they're in small cubes of a similar size. Melt a bit of butter or add a drizzle of oil to a heavy-bottomed saucepan. Season with salt and pepper.

Throw in the potatoes and onion, cover with a piece of grease-proof paper and put the lid on your pot.

Allow the vegetables to sweat over a low heat, stirring occasionally to ensure they're not sticking. If you feel they're going to stick and get burnt, add a few tablespoons of stock.

Once the onion and potatoes are soft but not coloured, pour in your stock. This can be homemade or from a stock cube.

Next add the rest of the chopped vegetables. If you don't like one of my suggestions, add something else (I'll give you some ideas for other combinations afterwards). Season once more with salt and pepper.

Bring to the boil and simmer until all the vegetables are soft.

Liquidise or blend until smooth. Shred and add the cooked chicken breast and blitz again for a short time.

If you like a clear soup with the vegetables left whole, that's perfect too.

I usually make large batches of soup and freeze it, so it's ready to defrost when I'm feeling low. Even if I can't eat anything else, I know I'm getting vegetables and protein and it's easy to digest.

Other flavours that I love combining are broccoli, sweet potato and toasted almonds; cauliflower and a pinch of turmeric; plain potato and leek; carrot and orange; mushroom with a dash of cream – the list and possibilities are endless. Simply make the base as above, and once the stock is poured in, add the flavour of your choice. It can be as simple or complex as you wish. If you're looking to put on a bit of weight or to make it all a little more luxurious, add a good dash of pouring cream once the soup is blended.

The most important thing is to season as you go along. That way the flavours will be brought out and you won't end up with a bland-tasting soup. Don't forget about fresh herbs and spices too. I often find I'm not able to stomach much spice, but something like freshly chopped coriander added to a carrot soup moments before you serve it can really make a wonderful addition. I tend not to add fresh herbs to soup that is going in the freezer, as the leaves tend to turn black. It's better to use them at the last minute, when you're ready to serve.

If nausea is really an issue, I always find it best to stick to dry foods such as toast or crackers. Again, once I've managed to eat a small amount, I'm usually able to carry on and eat a bit more. I find eating something like a few bread sticks, waiting for fifteen minutes and then trying a bowl of soup works. It's amazing how much better everything can be when you can eat a bit.

Only once have I been so ill that I couldn't stop vomiting and wasn't able to eat a morsel. It was awful and I'll never forget it. I found lying in a darkened room with a damp cloth over my eyes was the only relief I could get. At that time, I nibbled on sesame sticks. The saltiness and dryness was all I could manage. Needless to say, now I hate them!

I often ate seedless grapes. Even three or four can be enough to give you a bit of a lift and turn your complexion from green to normal.

Jelly sweets can be a good treat. I'm not ordinarily a fan of jellies, as I find them far too sweet and the flavours are not really what I enjoy. But, especially while I was on Cisplatin, I found they were one of the things I could stomach.

Another really odd thing I enjoyed even while I was feeling awful were individual trifles. Marks and Spencer do gorgeous ones and they were my little bit of indulgence. They also have fabulous fruit pots with things like melon and grapes and mango. Taken straight from the fridge they can be lovely, especially if your mouth is sore.

Body care

Something that would never have entered my mind when I began cancer treatment was how heightened my sense of smell would become. Just like during pregnancy, I find that I can be totally nauseated by certain smells. When you're feeling pretty pukey to begin with, getting into a hot shower and using a gel that smells sickly sweet isn't going to help.

When I went into hospital to have my mastectomy surgery, I had a bog-standard shower gel that was supposed to be grape flavoured. I will never forget how sick the sweet, cloying smell made me feel. It was also incredibly drying. So now I stick to really good ones with a fresh smell. It might sound crazy to spend money on shower gels but it's one of my indulgences that I know makes a difference to how I feel each morning. I don't spend massively on stuff I don't use but having a special shower gel is such a gorgeous treat. They also make wonderful presents for anyone who mightn't be well. Or, indeed, if you're totally healthy and want to feel great, you're allowed to have them too. It's a fabulous obsession and I recommend all of you try it!

I'm a massive fan of L'Occitane Citrus Verbena or Verveine shower gels. They're more expensive than supermarket ones but they last for ages and ages and are such a joy to use. Clarins do a delicious oil that can be put on after your shower. I used it when I was pregnant and, more recently, I've gotten back into the habit of smoothing it onto damp skin. It's a firming and toning body oil called Huile Tonic and it's packed with essential oils and is brilliant for avoiding stretch marks during pregnancy. Molton Brown do a divine shower gel called Black Peppercorn Body Wash and a more girly version called Pink Pepperpod, both of which are spicy and fresh rather than vomity sweet. Again, these last for ages and you only need a little dot in the palm of your hand each day.

I wasn't able to use many perfumes while sick. Many of the scents didn't smell the same and I found myself gagging. For a light and spritzy cologne, I love nothing more than Clarins Eau Dynamisante. This gorgeous scent comes in a spray as well as a body lotion and shower gel. My daughter steals this every time I buy it!

Probably the *grand dame* of all things delicious smelling has to be Jo Malone. We all know how stunning her products are and it's hard to go wrong with her scents. I am a devoted user of her Blackberry and Bay cologne. I could sniff it all day and think I might be slightly addicted to it. If you're looking for a special gift for a lady you love, knock yourself out and buy the body cream. Pomegranate Noir

Body Crème is utterly divine – I've given this as gifts to umpteen people who all adored it. As for her candles … If I ever win the Lotto, I'll have them in every room of my house!

For itchy skin, particularly burnt skin, I cannot find anything better than Aveeno with oatmeal – it is like a magic wand to irritated skin. It also comes in a handy pump dispenser.

Deodorant

Many women worry about using underarm deodorant, as there has been a lot of press about the harmful properties of some products. Again, it's always good to avoid anything with parabens. These harmful preservatives have been linked to breast cancer over the years. Many years ago I stopped using spray or roll-on deodorants from the supermarket and switched to ones made from natural ingredients. I'm not suggesting that one action will stop you from getting breast cancer – it certainly didn't work for me. But I feel it makes sense to avoid coating your underarm skin with chemicals each morning. Again, I've tried so many of these products I could open a stall. I find a lot of them useless. They seem to make me sweat and the smell from them is almost worse than BO! I've settled on a brand called Jason. They do shampoos and other products as well, but I find their deodorant sticks great. Dr Hauschka do some deodorants that are free of nasties also. Most pharmacies and health food shops carry a range of natural deodorants. The key is to find one that you can bear the smell of – most of them are herb based and it's a bit of a feat to avoid smelling like herb stuffing. Not the best odour in my book!

Skin care

There are so many incredible products on the market today that it's difficult to single them out. I've always maintained that once you find a skin-care system that suits your skin – stick to it.

I used a particular range of products for years and years but suddenly it began to cause irritation, so I tried and tested quite a few different ones.

I'm a Clarins girl all the way. I adore their products and they seem to suit my skin. The great news is that they use natural ingredients and essential oils so they smell great too. If I had to choose one item to buy from them it would be the Toning Lotion with Chamomile. Used on damp cotton wool, it is refreshing with the most beautiful, fresh smell. Their Double Serum is spectacular too. One of their most iconic products has to be Beauty Flash Balm. This is perfect for under make-up and works like a dream for skin looking a bit Princess Fiona-ish (green). Available online (www. clarins.com) and also in most department stores – the ladies at the counters there are trained to guide you.

Dr Hauschka, available in large department stores or health food shops, have a superb range of chemical-free products and I particularly love the Soothing Mask. Their lipsticks are beautiful too. They do lovely kits with mini-sized products that are perfect for travelling – or indeed for bringing to hospital. They cater for all skin types but I think where they really shine is for sensitive skin (www. drhauschka.com).

If you're suffering with break-outs and your skin is red and sore, the best thing to use is a bog-standard aqueous cream. This doubles up as a moisturiser and a soap substitute. It won't give you a kick, as it has no scent, but sometimes that's just what you need if you're feeling really nauseous. Available from chemists, it's cheap as chips.

Something that is wonderful to have, especially while in hospital, is a facial spray. The original one was by Evian and it's lovely, but a much cheaper version is Avène Thermal Spring Water spray. Either of these products is great to have to hand. They cool and refresh hot, parched facial skin without having to move from your bed!

La Roche-Posay have a wide range of products suitable for sensitive skin. Their sun-care products are particularly brilliant and can be used on small children. It's worth going into your local stockist's to speak to a trained member of staff to find which ones would work best for you. I adore their Sensitive Skin Micellar Solution – it removes all make-up, including mascara, and leaves the skin fresh without causing irritation (www.laroche-posay.ie).

If you're looking for all-natural, cruelty-free products with no chemicals, then Biofresh could be the one for you. Made with essential oils and phyto stem cells, they provide a wonderful way to treat your skin with the confidence that there are no nasties in there.

The range for acne is superb too. For more information go to www.
biofreshskincare.ie.

Another range of products that I've tried comes from Lindi Skin.
They have a specific range for chemotherapy patients, with all sorts of
goodies from face serum to soothing balm for dry and hands and feet.
There's a lovely pack called the Lindi Fight Back Pack which is a kit
containing sample sizes of their products. This makes a lovely gift for
someone or for yourself! Check them out at www.lindiskin.com.

E45 cream, just like aqueous cream, is one of those standard
moisturisers that can be used during radiation treatment too. I found
this particularly brilliant when used directly from the fridge. It's
cooling and is easily absorbed into burnt and parched skin. Even if
it's not going to set your world alight or make you feel as uplifted
as some of the more luxurious creams, it's a necessity if you're struggling with radiation burns, as there are very few products that I
found gentle enough when my skin was really raw. The marvellous
thing is that it's so cheap and can be bought in pharmacies or supermarkets. I used to stash tubs of it in my car, at my desk and around
my house. Each time I passed a tub I'd lather some on. That way
my skin didn't get overly tight and sore. It also helps massively with
the itching factor. It's a great practical one to have for lashing on,
while perhaps saving a nicer hand or foot lotion for the feel-good
factor!

Make-up
Even the least enthusiastic make-up wearers often tend to look for
help during cancer treatment. Suddenly you're faced with a no-
eyebrow situation, and perhaps your lashes have vamoosed too.
There's also the slightly green-tinged complexion and the often puffy
steroidinduced look.

All in all, it can be a good time to embrace make-up.

I happen to be a dedicated follower and wouldn't step outside the
house without my face on. But I've never felt the need for my
cosmetics more than when I'm at a particularly low ebb. I know it
can seem like a hassle to get out the make-up bag, but I cannot
express how much of a difference a little effort will make to how
you feel.

As I mentioned before, I love Clarins Beauty Flash Balm – I think every woman should own a tube of it! Yes, that's a sweeping statement but I will stand on a chair in the middle of my kitchen and hold my head high when I say it. This tube of deliciousness is perfect for under make-up and adds a glow that simply isn't there during cancer treatment. I use it every day without fail (www.clarins.com).

When it comes to foundation, I find that I need slightly more coverage during the 'green-faced' times. The best policy is to head to your nearest large department store and ask for a couple of samples. Skin tones vary so much and there is such a massive array of foundations on the market that it's really down to personal preference. I find Mac make-up hard to beat. They have something for everyone and their staff are so well trained. My advice is to visit your local Mac counter on a Monday morning or at a similar quiet time and they'll be willing and able to play with you. I've ended up practically having a makeover as they go through everything from eye shadows to foundation (www.maccosmetics.com).

Speaking of eye shadow, I find it's never a good look to use the pearlised pale shades. They might be nice on darker skins or during the summer months on pale folks such as me, but I found them draining while I was sick. So I experimented with some more robust colours. Browns are a good palate to stick to, as they add warmth to any skin tone and can be built on to create a more smoky or dramatic effect should that be required.

My favourite palate by far, and I've given many gifts of this to family and friends, is Urban Decay's Naked Eyeshadow Palette. There are several versions but the original one is a brilliant starting point. If, like me, you become addicted to their shadows you'll eventually end up with all of them! They have strong yet warm pigments and are easy to build up and apply. If you have the time and energy, Urban Decay run make-up classes. In my local House of Fraser they charge for the class but then you can redeem the full amount against products. So, essentially, the class is free. You also go home with a bag of goodies that you know how to apply. (www.urbandecay.com)

Lipstick can brighten up any jaded-looking face. I believe there should be lipstick police on each corner urging women to paint their pout! If you're looking for something moisturising and subtle,

I don't think you'll do better than Clinique Chubby Sticks. They're all about being moisturising in a kind and nourishing way and they don't taste awful! (www.clinique.com)

If you're looking for long-lasting and strong colours to really give your complexion a good lift, I've found nothing to stay on better than Rimmel Provocalips 16Hr Kissproof Lip Colour. This two-step system requires you to apply the colour followed by a sealing gloss coat. I have a bright pink and a siren red in this make and I love them both. (www.rimmellondon.com)

If you're suffering with badly chapped lips, my go-to product, which is also gorgeous to have in your holiday bag, comes from Guinot. This little tube will last ages and ages and is the most delicious and comforting thing I've ever found in a lip treatment. With avocado extract and shea butter, it's light and easily absorbed and there's no gag factor, nor do I feel like I'm coated in petroleum jelly. Baume Lèvres Confort Lip Balm would also make for a perfect gift while visiting someone in hospital.

Bronzers can be a minefield, especially when your colour is compromised. Having tried a ton of different ones I have stuck with the Duo Bronzer from TanOrganic. Eco-certified, this is made with natural ingredients and has a brilliant knack of looking good on all skin types. My daughter, who is sallow, steals mine and it's just as good on her skin. (www.tanorganic.com)

The write stuff
My next tip is the one that has been my saviour. Above all else, writing has been the perfect therapy for me over the years. I began writing my first novel, *Designer Genes*, from a hospital bed. That was eight years ago and to date I have had eleven books published! I don't expect everyone to drop everything and become an author by next week. But I cannot stress how incredibly cathartic it is to write your thoughts down. Once they're out of your head and on paper or in a computer, it's as if the worries or woes have been removed. Nobody needs to read your words if you don't want them to. You can go for a diary format for a more therapeutic method. A diary obviously has a small space for each day, so you don't have to write much. As the days fill up you can see your progress, which can be

deeply satisfying. Many people swear by a gratitude diary, where you list the things that you feel grateful for.

Or perhaps start off by buying a pretty little notebook that will entice you into filling it. There's no right or wrong way of writing so it's a win-win situation. Pour your heart out and I bet you'll feel relieved afterwards.

What to Pack in a Hospital Bag When Having a Mastectomy

This is something that I learned the hard way. The first time I went to hospital (apart from giving birth) was to have a bi-lateral mastectomy. I brought half the house with me and most of it was wrong. So I've drawn up a little list of the essentials that I actually needed.

- Pyjamas that button up the front – your arms will be compromised and you may have a drain in place so T-shirt-style tops are no use.
- Earplugs – hospitals are noisy all the time. Little yellow spongy plugs can mean the difference between a night's sleep or being constantly and frustratingly woken.
- Eye mask – preferably one with a thin elastic strap rather than one that is tied in a bow. You will probably end up sleeping on your back to avoid hurting your wound so a thick bow isn't comfortable to sleep on.
- Facial wipes – there are so many on the market now that it's easy to find ones that don't cause irritation. If you can't get out of bed, these are wonderful for a quick freshen up.
- A hairbrush with a long handle – it's not easy to brush your hair for a few days after a mastectomy, especially if it's a double mastectomy. A brush with a longer handle makes things so much easier.
- Post-surgery bra – I didn't know about these at the time but I'd recommend investing in one (www.theyahealthcare.com).
- Facial spray – to help you feel refreshed.
- Flip-flops – especially if you are going to be in a ward. You'll be glad of them if you want to shower in a communal bathroom.

- Lightweight dressing gown – hospitals are notoriously hot places so a dressing gown is only necessary to preserve your dignity if you need to walk about rather than for warmth.
- Audible app – this fabulous little app allows you to listen to books on your phone or tablet. Often, especially after surgery, it's difficult to concentrate on reading, so, with this downloaded to your device, you can simply listen to the stories. (www.audible.co.uk)
- Earphones – for listening to books or music. Without meaning to sound horrible, they can also be fantastic if you want to avoid long, exhausting conversations with people you don't know!

Questions I Want to Ask but I'm Afraid to Sound Silly

Q: What is cancer?

(We're all supposed to know the answer to this, right?)

A: We all have cancer cells floating around our bodies. But when those cancer cells begin to grow in an uncontrolled manner and produce abnormal cells in the body, problems arise. The disease of cancer develops when the body's normal control mechanism stops working.

Q: What are tumours?

(It's such a horrible word.)

A: When old cancer cells fail to die off in the body they grow out of control, forming new, abnormal cells. These clumps of cells form a mass of tissue called a tumour.

Some cancers, such as leukaemia (cancer of the blood) don't form tumours.

Tumours can present as lumps that feel foreign to the body.

Q: Do the lumps hurt?

(I remember hearing an old wives' tale that if a lump hurt it couldn't be cancer. That's rubbish.)

A: Sometimes they do and sometimes they don't. It really depends on where they are. In my case, my tumours have been around my neck, shoulders, head and upper chest. When pressed, most of them caused me pain.

Q: Is there always a lump if a woman has breast cancer?

(Most people don't know there are other signs to watch out for.)

A: Absolutely not. There can be puckering of the skin or mottled skin that looks like orange peel. The nipple can be inverted. One breast can be slightly bigger than the other (when it wasn't before). There could be a discharge from the nipple.

Q: What is a fine-needle biopsy?

A: This is very often the first port of call when a lump is discovered in easily accessible tissue such as the breast or neck. Local anaesthetic is injected into the site. A thin needle is inserted and some of the suspect cells are removed and sent to pathology to be tested for cancer.

Q: What is a CT scan?

A: CT stands for computerised tomography. The CT machine uses X-ray images taken from different angles while using computer processing to create cross-sectioned pictures in a slice-by-slice method to show every bit of our bodies from our bones through blood vessels and soft tissue inside.

During a CT scan the person must lie very still on a bed. This is to avoid blurring the images. You will be asked to take a breath and hold it for a few seconds at a time. The table will move through a large dome-shaped scanner. There'll be a whirring sound, but it's not scary or painful.

Contrast is most commonly injected through a cannula (small needle in your arm). It helps to give a clearer picture of what's going on inside your body.

The contrast causes a short but, in my experience, not unpleasant sensation. There's a rush of heat and a slight metallic taste at the back of the throat, followed by a similar sensation in the bladder. Some people report a feeling of needing to pee. But this doesn't last long.

Q: What exactly is chemotherapy?

(For the record, I thought it might involve a large machine and possibly a tunnel.)

A: Chemotherapy is cancer medicine that comes in either tablet or liquid form. It's usually administered by a drip using a needle in your hand (a cannula). So for all the world, it's a bag of cancer-slaying liquid that gets hung on a pole and drip-fed into your vein.

Q: What do I do when I'm having chemotherapy?

(I had visions of dry ice circulating the room and invasive probes.)

A: You sit in a chair or lie on a bed. The nurse puts a cannula or needle in the back of your hand and the chemotherapy slowly drizzles into your vein. It's a long and boring process but not scary. You might feel sleepy due to the anti-nausea drugs you are given at the same time. So you'll probably have a little snooze.

Q: Will I definitely vomit after it?

(My image of a chemotherapy patient involved a person hugging a toilet indefinitely.)

A: There is no need to be violently ill nowadays. There are amazing anti-nausea medications on the market, but you must tell your doctor if you feel sick. Over my ten diagnoses I have never vomited due to chemotherapy.

Q: Will my hair fall out immediately?

(I thought I'd be bald by the time I got home the first night.)

A: No, not necessarily. Some chemotherapy medicines don't cause alopecia at all while others only cause thinning. But if you stand to lose all your hair, it can go any time from three weeks after the first treatment. But it won't fall out in one go. It happens gradually. It won't leave your head and fall on the floor like a small furry animal.

Q: Will *all* my hair fall out?

(I was hoping for annoying body hair to go first.)

A: As luck would have it, all body hair and pubic hair goes bar the hair on your legs. How unfair is that? It will mean no bikini-line waxing or underarm shaving but why, oh why, doesn't leg hair go too? Eyebrows and even eyelashes can be lost, but not always. I only lost my lashes once and they grew back swiftly.

Q: Does radiotherapy hurt?

(This does involve a massive machine with a flying saucer so I instantly feared it.)

A: In general, the actual radiotherapy causes no pain. You lie on a bed and the machine doesn't actually touch you. It's a lot like having an X-ray. Unless the tumour is somewhere extremely sensitive, such as the back of the head, it shouldn't cause more than mild skin burn. There are also some types of internal radiotherapy, which are more invasive. But for most patients, it is a painless process.

Q: Will radiotherapy make me sick?

(I assumed it would, seeing as it's carried out every day.)

A: Radiotherapy causes fatigue and the effect is cumulative, so the tiredness builds up over time. But in my experience it didn't make me actually sick.

Q: Is it best to take to my bed during radiotherapy or chemotherapy?

(I dreaded the thought of being bed-bound for weeks on end.)

A: While it's always good to conserve energy during cancer treatment, I have found regular exercise vital. It can be the last thing you feel like doing but it really helps to build energy! Most people have a couple of 'down days' during chemotherapy where they feel more tired and sick than usual, but this passes.

Q: Can I exercise during cancer treatment?

(I would love nothing more than the answer to be a strict no to this question as I'm so lazy!)

A: I know from experience that exercise is completely vital during treatment. The best way to avoid fatigue, sickness and whole host of problems is to get up and move. It's not what you'll feel like some of the time, but even a five-minute walk in the fresh air will help – I promise.

Q: Can I wear make-up or fake tan ever again?

(I don't go out in public without make-up and feared I'd be banished to the darkness during treatment!)

A: Yes, of course you can still use your beauty products. In fact, I think it's doubly important to feel as good as you can. There are lots of organic or paraben-free products on the market now so there's no need to go bare faced even if you worry about chemicals. Lipstick on and let's get going!

Q: Will I have diarrhoea all the time?

(I genuinely considered buying a packet of Pull-Ups prior to my first chemotherapy.)

A: Hearsay had me believing I'd be either leaning into the loo or sitting on it for my entire treatment time. I even thought about having the bathroom done up beforehand, as I was planning on spending so much time in there. But side effects are different with every patient. Personally, my bowel thinks it's a skip while I'm on treatment and I suffer with dreadful constipation. But again, there is medication to help with diarrhoea or constipation.

Q: Will I be exhausted and half-asleep all the time?

(I'd decided I would be like a zombie for six months.)

A: Although there will be days when you feel really tired, many patients also suffer with insomnia. Regular exercise helps with this.

Q: Will everyone I meet, even strangers, know I'm a cancer patient by looking at me?

(I thought I'd look totally different and incredibly ill.)

A: I chose to wear a wig so my head looked 'normal'. I also wore make-up and, of course, my usual clothes. Unless I told them, people who didn't know me had no idea I was a cancer patient. It's possible to be a vixen not a victim.

Q: How long does it take the hair to grow back once treatment is over?

(I assumed it would take months to even start.)

A: Almost as soon as the treatment ends it's as if your hair has been waiting in the wings to spring into action. In some rare cases the hair doesn't return. But for most people it's very quick. It took a good eighteen months for my hair to have a proper style again, but I was pleasantly surprised by how swiftly I could ditch my wig.

Q: Will my hair look the same as before when it starts to grow?

(I'm blonde with poker-straight hair. I assumed the new hair would be the same!)

A: In a word – no. Your hair won't look anything like before at first. It will be curly and either dark or grey! I looked like a baby monkey for a while, but as it grew the colour lightened and it became straight.

Q: Do I have to keep shaving my hair to strengthen it?
(I was told this by so many people.)
A: I would've sobbed like a baby if anyone had shaved my head as soon as my new hair had sprouted. I simply let mine grow and, in time, had it trimmed regularly. I know it probably would've made my hair stronger to shave it but I couldn't bear it. I wanted it to grow!

Q: Can I use normal dye on my new hair?
(I was told umpteen times that I couldn't.)
A: The first time I lost my hair, I endured dark curls and looked like a Monchhichi monkey from the eighties for a while. I assumed the only option was a vegetable dye. It was about as effective as food colouring. I found a hairdresser who agreed to use a non-peroxide colour. It lifted my spirits higher than a bag of ecstasy and my hair didn't fall out or break off, nor did my scalp disintegrate or bubble up in blisters. Result!

Q: If I follow a special diet will it cure my cancer?
(I know this is a contentious issue ...)
A: I have tried many diets over the years. I gave up dairy, wheat, sugar, alcohol and smiling. The smiling disappeared organically along with the exclusion diets. None of this worked for me. As far as I know, there is no medical evidence that diet alone can cure cancer. Obviously it's important to eat a healthy, balanced diet – but that's just common sense, right?

Q: I feel like a junkie! Should I stop some of the tablets I'm on? I never wanted to take this much medication?
(There were times when I feared I would rattle as I walked I was on so many tablets ...)
A: Try to keep in mind that all the drug taking will probably be transient. For most cancer patients, treatments only last a matter of

months. Anti-nausea drugs, painkillers, sleeping tablets, anti-anxiety tablets, laxatives, diarrhoea tablets or whatever you need to take were invented for a reason. If you take them when you are in dire need, they'll work and you will have a better quality of life while on treatment. There are no medals for vomiting more, being in pain or not being able to sleep.

Q: Can I take alternative medicines alongside my chemotherapy or radiotherapy?

(I did this, so I am speaking from experience here ...)

A: Please do not ingest anything without clearing it with your doctor first. At one point I was happily taking Chinese herbal medicine, assuming it was helping my body to fight. At the time I had both cancer and an autoimmune disease. It turned out the substance I was taking was actually coating my cells and would have prevented the chemotherapy from working. It terrified me and it was a lesson well learned.

Q: Can I have facials during chemotherapy?

(I love the relaxing feeling of a facial, and during treatment it can be the ultimate treat.)

A: In some cases it's safe to have a facial. But for many people with breast cancer, or indeed head or neck cancer, facials might not be a good plan. During a facial the therapist uses massage – this moves lymph around the face, neck and décolletage. If there is cancer present in the lymph nodes, this is a bad idea. We don't need infected lymph nodes being stimulated or moved. So ask your medical team before making an appointment. Try reflexology instead – this is definitely safe.

Q: I read stuff online and it's not what my doctor said. Who should I believe?

(I hold my hands up here – I am guilty of hitting Google, especially when I'm worried.)

A: Remember every case of cancer is different. The only people who can answer your questions are your doctors and nurses.

Q: Is it OK to laugh during treatment?

(I genuinely worried about this in the beginning!)

A: I have always had a dark sense of humour and, believe me, it grew legs when I started my fight. Laughter is the best medicine, right? So go for it and never forget you are still you. Don't allow cancer to change that.

Q: Can I drink alcohol while I'm having treatment?

(I assumed it was a total no-no!)

A: Again, depending on the type of cancer involved, most doctors allow patients to drink in moderation. If I'm out for a meal or at a special occasion, I will absolutely enjoy a drink. Check it out with your medical team, but generally speaking it's not a problem. I can't drink much any more, as it makes me feel too sick and I get a headache. But I'm all for doing things in moderation if they make you happy!

Q: Will I ever feel normal again?

(This was probably my biggest fear …)

A: I was and still am astounded by how my body bounces back after each round of treatment. When I was in the wars I worried that I would never be 'me' again. But I'm always astonished by how my body has regenerated. As the years have progressed it takes me longer each time. But life can and does return to normal.

Q: I worry constantly about recurrence. Is that normal?

(If I had a euro for each time I'm asked this, I'd be very rich.)

I'm probably not the best person to ask about this. I haven't ever gone for too long without being diagnosed again. But don't forget I have a cancer gene, so I'm predisposed to the disease. Anyone who has been through cancer is going to worry. Sadly, that's unavoidable. But once you are looking after yourself and eating sensibly and taking a bit of exercise and trying to be healthy, that's all you can do. Go for regular check-ups and, as the years pass by, you'll grow in confidence that the cancer (hopefully) won't return.

Acknowledgements

Being afforded the honour of having my work published over the last few years has given me a high I will never come down from. *Talk to the Headscarf* is slightly different, in so far as it's my own story with no makey-uppy bits. Thank you to my agent Sheila Crowley of Curtis Brown for all your encouragement and for suggesting I write this memoir. You are and always will be a shining star in my sky.

Thanks to Breda, Jim, Joanna, Bernard, Ruth and Siobhan at Hachette Ireland for helping and believing in me all these years. Huge thanks to my editor Ciara Doorley for your positive and warm guidance and to Hazel for your copy editing. For the second edition of this book I had the wonderful Sherise Hobbs from Headline UK adding her backup. Thanks also to Emma Dunne for your copy editing skills and to Seán Costello for your brilliant proofreading. I have such an amazing team behind me and I am so grateful to each one of you. Thanks to Emily Quinn for the fun photo shoot and I am still mortified at being so damn late. I will never listen to that satnav again. She's a liar.

I have the best family on the planet! Firstly, let's hear it for my hubby Cian and our two cherished children, Sacha and Kim. You three are my lifeblood and the best incentive I have to keep fighting the good fight. You make me whole and I am blessed every day of my life to have you by my side.

My parents have nurtured, loved and encouraged me always. Despite my vomiting in the flowerbeds after a fill of vodka, aged fourteen (and many other similar scenarios), not to mention my talented ability to attract cancer, you've never lost faith in me. I hope the anxiety and worry might be somewhat cancelled out by making myself useful writing books. Thank you for instilling in me the hell-raiser instinct that has gotten me through the darker moments. My strength is a direct result of your unconditional love and faith.

Thank you to my brother Tim and his partner Hilary; Robyn and her husband Joe; Steffy, her hubby Stan and daughter Camille for being the best family a gal could wish for. Nobody outside the 'inner circle' could possibly evoke such Monty Python-esque conversations. Thank you all for the wine-spurting-out-my-nose belly laughs and the sheer irreverence with which you all conduct yourselves.

Thanks to the McGraths for all your support.

Huge thanks to the amazing friends I've met along the way. So many laughs, so much dancing, tons of support, knowing you've got my back. We've all come a long way together. I would be lost without you all.

Now I come to my medical team. The people who have literally used their expertise, kindness and tireless dedication to help me beat cancer ten times. Dr Callaghan Condon was my stepping-stone to a medical system that has saved my life. He tapped me into a nest of incredible medical superstars. The first day I walked into your office, you saved me. Thank you, Cal.

Dr Frances Stafford is the lady who daintily danced on the grave of my crippling autoimmune disease – dermatomyositis. A hideous condition with an unfortunately long name, but it didn't stand a chance once Frances took the reins. Thank you from the bottom of my heart.

My special thanks to Dr Michael Moriarty for helping me with his vast radiology knowledge. He is one of life's true gentlemen. I hope he is enjoying his retirement. Big thanks to all the radiology team in St Vincent's Private Hospital for zapping me and frying those nasty nodes! When I first saw Professor Armstrong speaking at a medical conference I knew I would ask for him should I require more radiation. He is so knowledgeable and precise I knew he would look after me. I've darkened his door many times and he has been amazing. Thank you, Professor Armstrong.

Dr David Fennelly is my oncologist and most definitely my hero. Nothing can repay his care and unbending knowledge and the confidence he has instilled in me from day one. David is so approachable and easy to talk to, he removes the fear I might otherwise have had of cancer. He has never flinched or sprinted in the other direction when he has seen me coming up the corridor towards him. At this stage, David and his team must've had moments, while looking at my ever-expanding file, when they pondered sending me to the vet to be put down. David, I am humbled and grateful beyond words for everything you do for me, and all your patients. Thank you sounds so feeble.

To all the front-desk ladies, not forgetting Michael, at Blackrock Clinic. I haven't named you all, for fear I might omit a name and cause offence – thank you for greeting me with a smile and a chat every time I come in. The difference your warmth makes is vast. To the nursing staff of the Fitzgerald and Nightingale Units, thank you for caring for me so kindly each and every time I've come for sleepovers. Special thanks to all the nurses and staff of the Oncology day unit for making my frequent visits so pleasant.

Singled out thanks must go to Liz for bringing me cups of real coffee. My only gripe with the Oncology day unit is the coffee.

Blackrock Clinic is known as 'Hotel Blackrock' in our house. I can't say I would recommend going to hospital for a holiday, but if you have to go somewhere, you'll find it damn hard to find a better place. Thank you all for keeping me alive.

Thanks to all my 'mum' friends at St Gerard's School for helping and being so kind over the past ten years. There were days that I quite simply couldn't have done without you. A lift home from school or an offer to take the kids to a party meant more than you will ever know. Thanks to Tom Geraghty, headmaster of the senior school, and Dr Deirdre Farrell, headmistress of the junior school, for your background support over the years. Community is such an important thing and I was blessed to be in the centre of an amazing example of this.

Huge thanks to Brian Moore and the staff of Rathdown School for welcoming and looking after Kim.

Special thanks to Tom. I know you won't ever read this, firstly because you're a cat and too busy sleeping on a pile of freshly ironed laundry. But you de-stress me with your purrs and blinks as I watch you dozing. You prove that being fat, furry and stripy is where it's at. When I grow up, if I can't be a fairy, I want to be you.

Thanks also to Herbie-doodle. When Cian came home with a puppy without asking me I honestly didn't know what to think. But you've won my heart and the hearts of all the family. You accompany me on my many walks with Mum and make us both realise that life is all about smiling and burying slices of toast.

Heartfelt thanks to Marie Robinson who has been a wonderful friend and fuss-free help for so many years. I can't begin to name the amount of times you came in and knew exactly what needed doing.

Finally I want to thank all the amazing people who've bought my books so far. Without readers I couldn't continue with this job, so thank you all for making my dream of being a writer come true. Thank you all for engaging with me on Facebook (Author Emma Hannigan) and Twitter (@MsEmmaHannigan) or for sending emails via my contact page on my website (www.emmahannigan.com). I hope that by sharing my experience you might realise that there is always hope and that there can be life during and after cancer.